D1556134

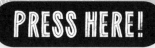

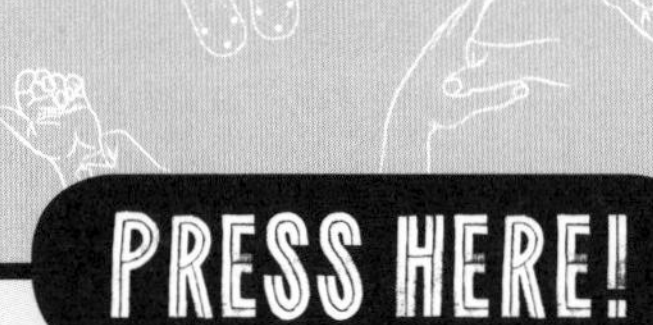

ACUPRESSURE

~FOR BEGINNERS~

PRESS HERE!

ACUPRESSURE

~FOR BEGINNERS~

HOW TO RELEASE AND BALANCE ENERGY FLOW

BOB DOTO

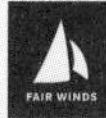

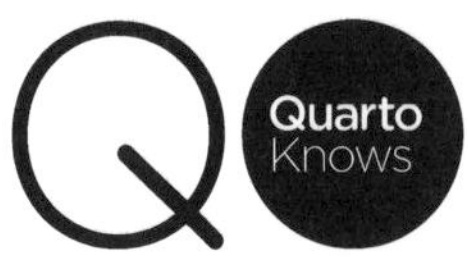

Inspiring | Educating | Creating | Entertaining

First Published in 2019 by Fair Winds Press, an imprint of The Quarto Group.

100 Cummings Center, Suite 265-D, Beverly, MA 01915, USA. T (978) 282-9590 F (978) 283-2742

23 22 21 20 19 1 2 3 4 5

ISBN: 978-1-59233-871-9

Digital edition published in 2019

QUAR.307050

Conceived, edited, and designed by Quarto Publishing plc. 6 Blundell Street, London N7 9BH

Editor: Claire Waite Brown
Senior art editor: Emma Clayton
Designer: Joanna Bettles
Illustrator: Kuo Kang Chen
Publisher: Samantha Warrington

Printed in China

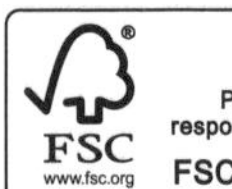

MIX
Paper from responsible sources
FSC® C104723

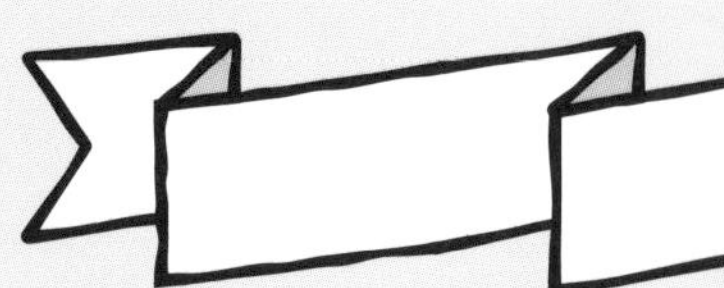

Chapter 1

Chapter 2

CONTENTS

WELCOME

MY FIRST EXPERIENCE OF ACUPRESSURE CAME NOT IN A MASSAGE SESSION, BUT RATHER IN A YOGA CLASS. THAT DAY I HAD BEEN EXPERIENCING SOME KNEE PAIN WHILE LEARNING A NEW POSTURE. AFTER CLASS I MENTIONED THIS TO MY TEACHER, WHO HAD ME LIE DOWN ON MY BACK. HE TOOK OUT A STRONG, MEDICINAL-SMELLING OINTMENT AND BEGAN TO RUB IT ON A POINT ABOUT A HAND'S WIDTH BELOW MY KNEE, WHERE HE APPLIED PRESSURE FOR ABOUT THREE MINUTES. WHEN I GOT UP AND REALIZED THAT MY PAIN HAD DISSIPATED BY ABOUT 75 PERCENT, I KNEW I HAD TO LEARN THIS TECHNIQUE.

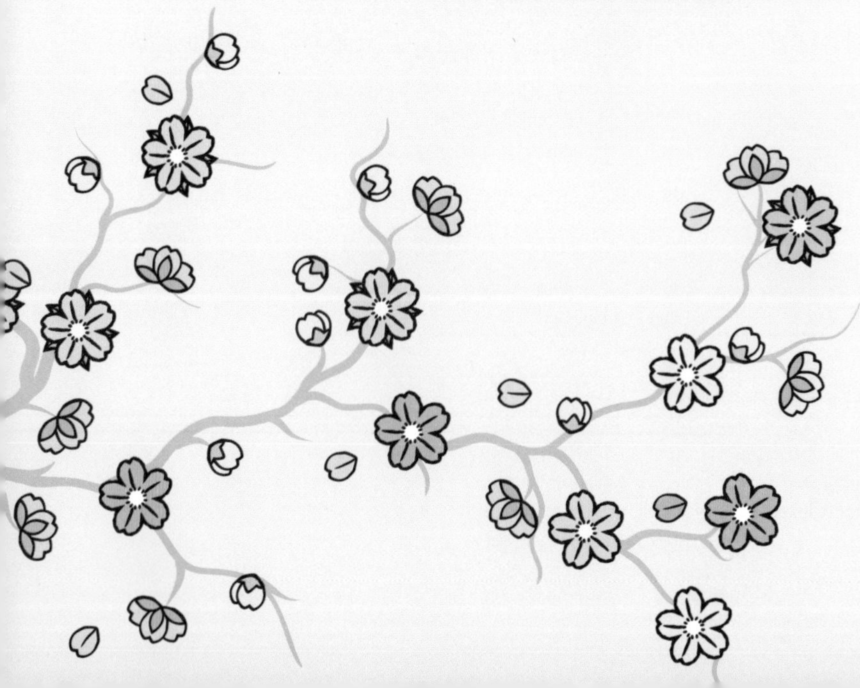

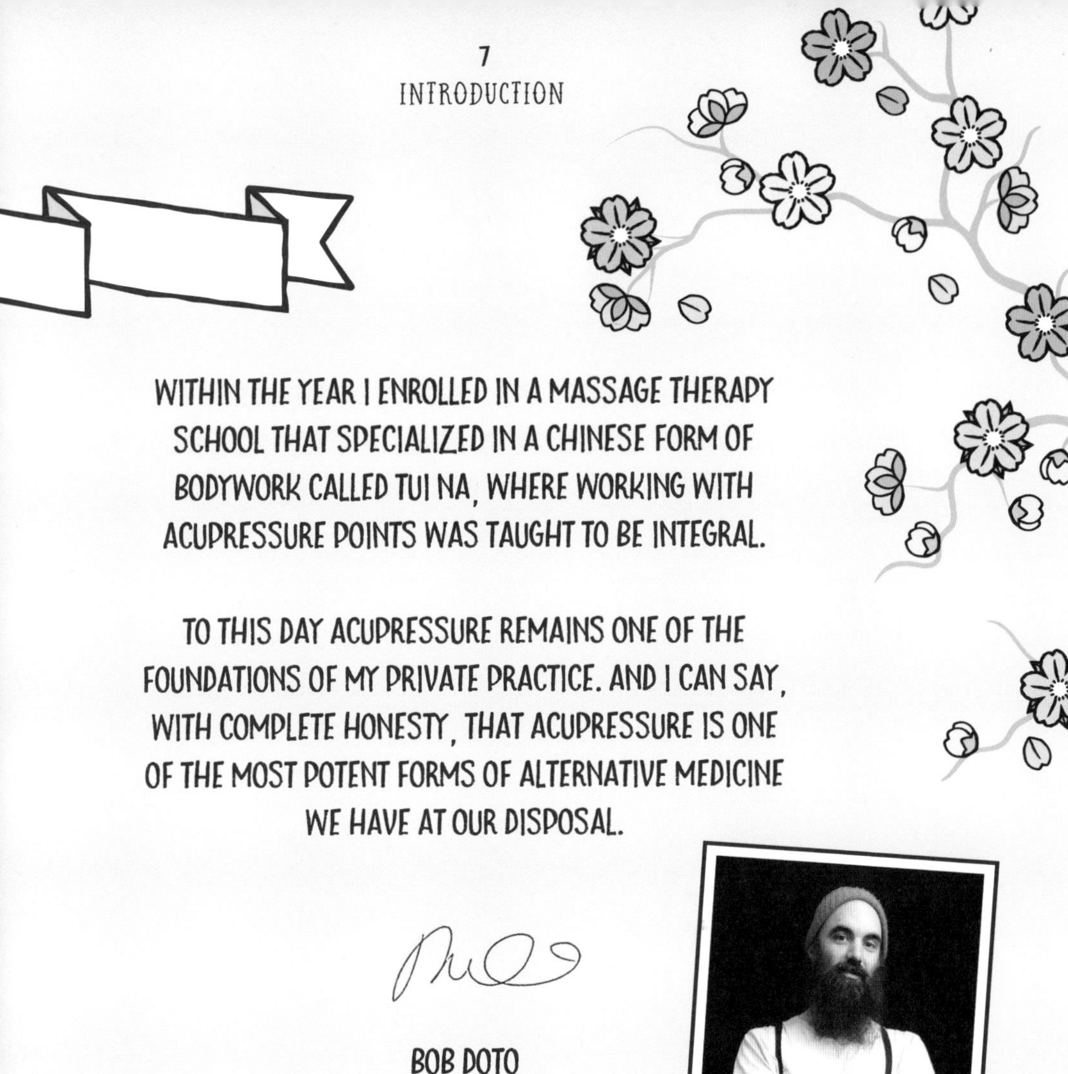

WITHIN THE YEAR I ENROLLED IN A MASSAGE THERAPY SCHOOL THAT SPECIALIZED IN A CHINESE FORM OF BODYWORK CALLED TUI NA, WHERE WORKING WITH ACUPRESSURE POINTS WAS TAUGHT TO BE INTEGRAL.

TO THIS DAY ACUPRESSURE REMAINS ONE OF THE FOUNDATIONS OF MY PRIVATE PRACTICE. AND I CAN SAY, WITH COMPLETE HONESTY, THAT ACUPRESSURE IS ONE OF THE MOST POTENT FORMS OF ALTERNATIVE MEDICINE WE HAVE AT OUR DISPOSAL.

BOB DOTO

DISCLAIMER

The information presented in this book is not intended as a substitute for training by a licensed acupressure instructor. The methodologies and protocol presented here should only be utilized as a gift to the readers themselves and to their loved ones. If you are inspired by what you learn here, you are encouraged to join an accredited acupressure therapy course.

ABOUT THIS BOOK

1

Preliminary Concepts

PAGES 10-21

This chapter looks at fundamental concepts associated with acupressure. Starting with a discussion of one of the most elusive of these, "qi," you will develop a basic understanding of the meridians through which qi travels, ultimately arriving at an understanding of the acupoint itself.

2

Guidelines and Approaches

PAGES 22-35

This chapter considers the anatomy of the hands and how to use them to work on acupoints. The guidelines discuss how much pressure to apply and the various sensations you might feel in an acupressure treatment.

3

The Points

PAGES 36-87

This chapter provides an in-depth overview of the 50 points used for the treatments in the following chapter. Each point discussed will include the English translation to the traditional Chinese name, a description of its anatomical location, the conditions for which it is commonly used, as well as any interesting notes worth mentioning.

NAMES
THE ABBREVIATED NAME RELATES TO THE MERIDIAN THE POINT LIES ON

LOCATION
THIS TEXT GIVES A DETAILED DESCRIPTION OF WHERE TO FIND THE POINT

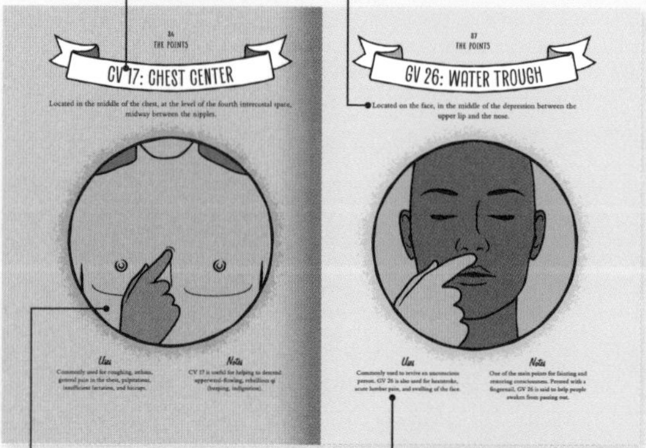

LOCATION ARTWORK
ARTWORKS ILLUSTRATE WHERE TO FIND THE POINT

USES
POINTS HAVE MANY USES, AND THE MOST COMMON ONES ARE DETAILED HERE

Treatment Plans

PAGES 88-116

This chapter details some common conditions and the points you can concentrate on to ease them, with advice for some extra self-care approaches that may help.

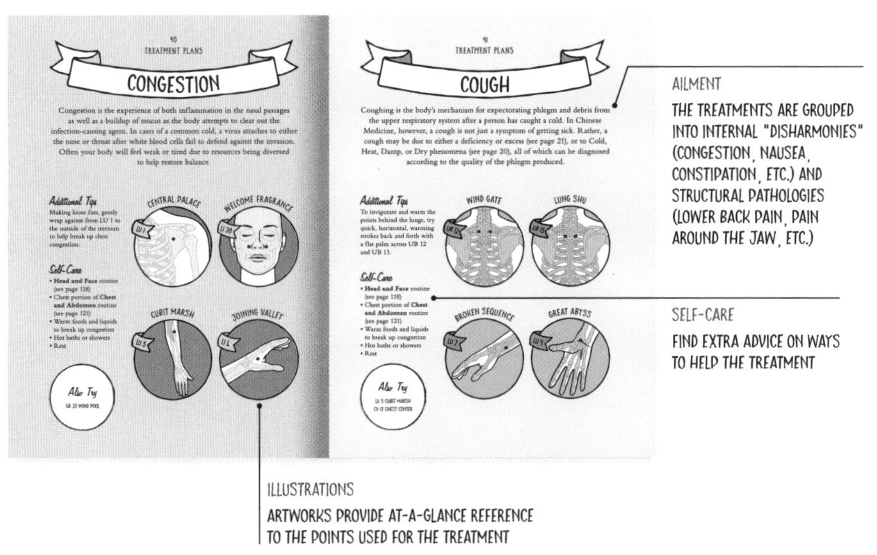

CONGESTION
COUGH
AILMENT
THE TREATMENTS ARE GROUPED INTO INTERNAL "DISHARMONIES" (CONGESTION, NAUSEA, CONSTIPATION, ETC.) AND STRUCTURAL PATHOLOGIES (LOWER BACK PAIN, PAIN AROUND THE JAW, ETC.)
SELF-CARE
FIND EXTRA ADVICE ON WAYS TO HELP THE TREATMENT
ILLUSTRATIONS
ARTWORKS PROVIDE AT-A-GLANCE REFERENCE TO THE POINTS USED FOR THE TREATMENT

The Routines

PAGES 117-123

This chapter details how to apply the self-care protocols referred to in the previous chapter.

Points Index

PAGES 124-125

The points and their page numbers are listed here in alphabetical order, to provide an easy reference when using the treatment plans.

1 PRELIMINARY CONCEPTS

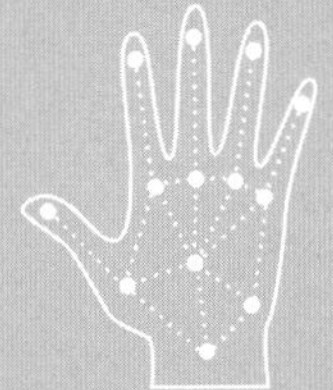

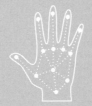

When there is no movement there is pain.
When there is movement there is no pain.

TRADITIONAL CHINESE SAYING

WHAT IS QI?

In the popular mind, **qi** is often thought of as something mysterious, mystical, or even spooky. But, in reality, while certainly a slippery idea, qi is far more accessible a concept.

The Chinese character for "qi" is depicted by the characters for steam and rice, which tells us a great deal about its nature. At one level steam and rice signify both the material and immaterial qualities of qi. Qi can be something we manipulate through **touch**, like rice, or it can **move** of its own accord, like steam, acting more as a motivator than something that is motivated.

As a substance, qi is able to be directed. Skilled hands can push qi into different areas of the body that may need more vitality. A practitioner can **invigorate** static qi, **calm** excited qi, and **gather** or **disperse** qi depending on what will better serve the receiver.

When thought of in its more formless, immaterial state, qi acts as a **life force**. It's in understanding this that we see qi as the motivating force behind all of our body's functions. Specifically, qi is known to:

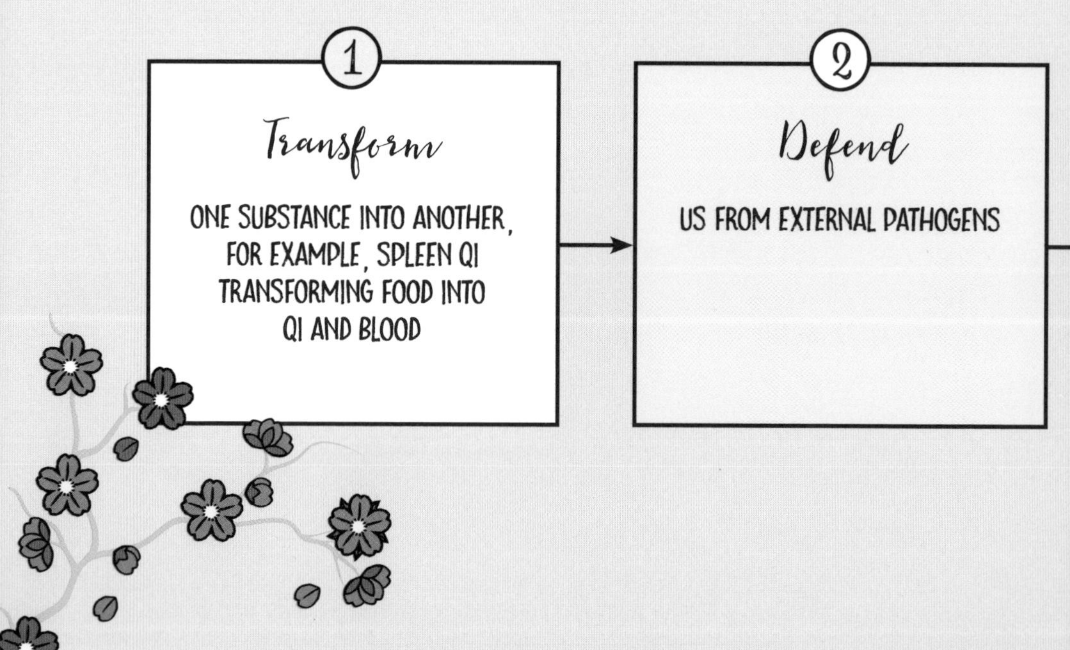

1
Transform
ONE SUBSTANCE INTO ANOTHER, FOR EXAMPLE, SPLEEN QI TRANSFORMING FOOD INTO QI AND BLOOD
2
Defend
US FROM EXTERNAL PATHOGENS

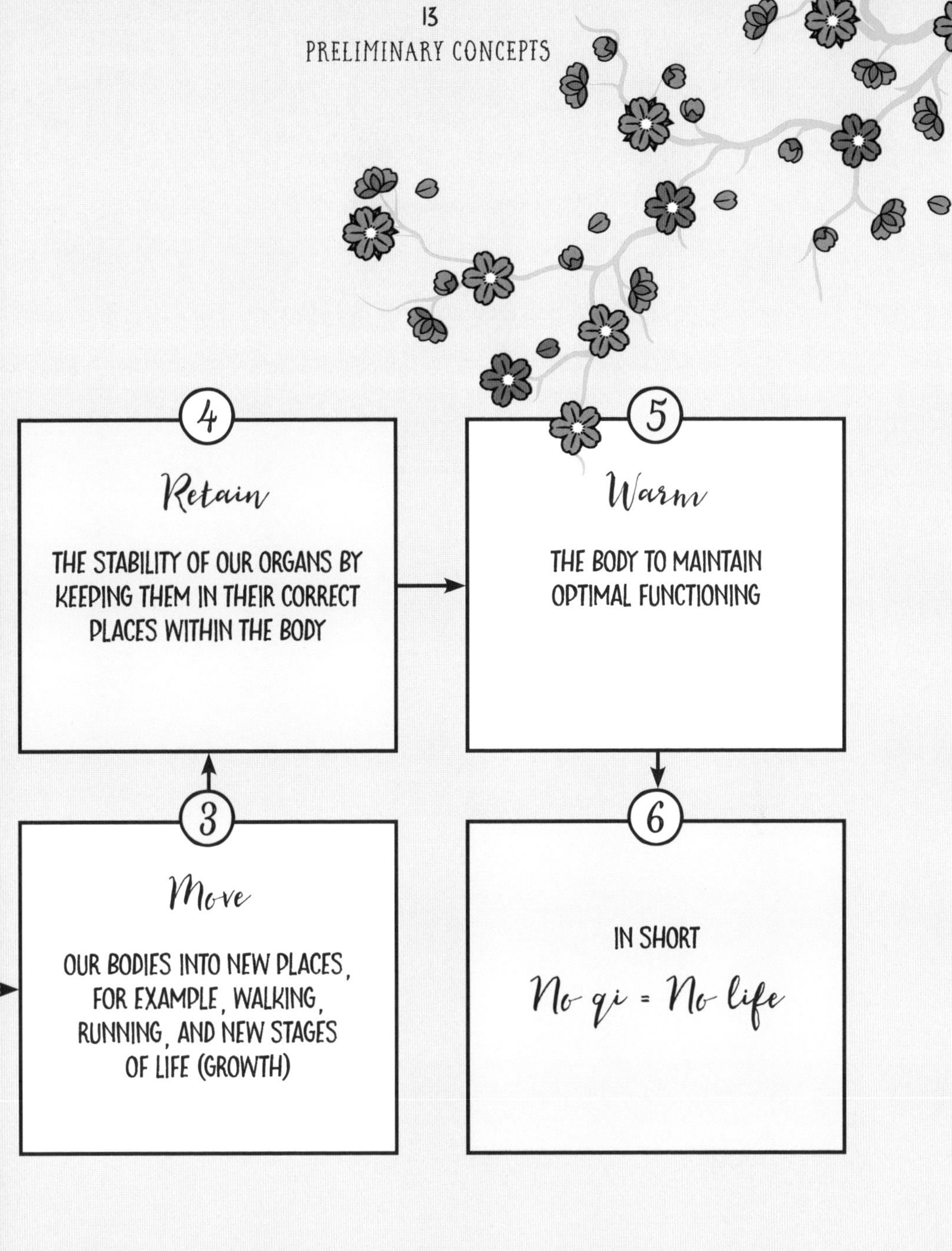
4
Retain
THE STABILITY OF OUR ORGANS BY KEEPING THEM IN THEIR CORRECT PLACES WITHIN THE BODY
5
Warm
THE BODY TO MAINTAIN OPTIMAL FUNCTIONING
3
Move
OUR BODIES INTO NEW PLACES, FOR EXAMPLE, WALKING, RUNNING, AND NEW STAGES OF LIFE (GROWTH)
6
IN SHORT
No qi = No life

WHAT IS A MERIDIAN?

If **qi** can be moved, then surely it must have places to go and ways of getting there. A **meridian**, sometimes called a channel, acts like a highway along which qi travels. There are 20 of these throughways of qi, the most common of which are the 12 **principal meridians** (named after certain organs in the body) and two **extraordinary meridians** (named after significant functions).

Principal Meridians

LUNG (LU)

LARGE INTESTINE (LI)

STOMACH (ST)

SPLEEN (SP)

HEART (HT)

SMALL INTESTINE (SI)

BLADDER (UB)

KIDNEY (KD)

PERICARDIUM (PC)

SAN JIAO (SJ)

GALL BLADDER (GB)

LIVER (LV)

Extraordinary Meridians

GOVERNING VESSEL (GV)

CONCEPTION VESSEL (CV)

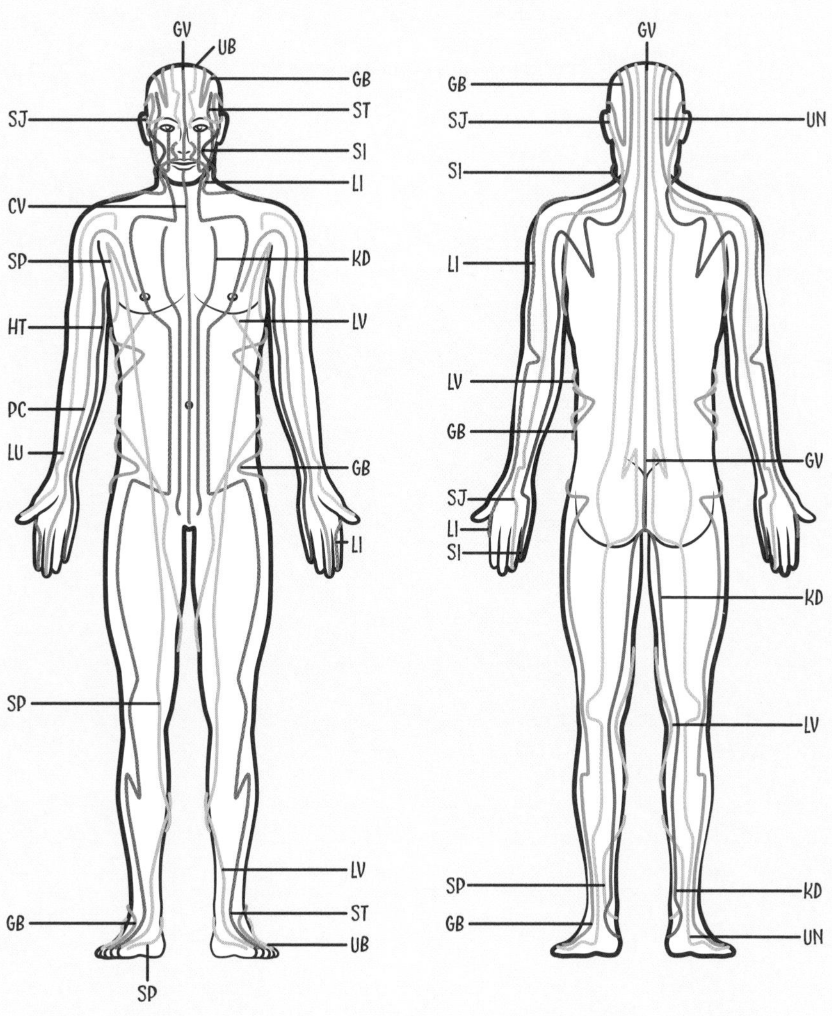

By gravitating to certain avenues of energetic flow, **qi** has done us a great service. **Meridians** provide practitioners with a blueprint or map of **energetic movement** throughout the body, which allows us to visualize where exactly the body may not be functioning properly due to stasis in the channels, and how and where we might try to **move** or **break up** this **congestion**.

WHAT IS AN ACUPOINT?

An **acupoint** is an area of concentrated **qi**, or "point," along a given **meridian**. When the qi in these points stops moving or becomes "stagnated," the points and the surrounding tissue can be manipulated in order to get things going again.

Acupoints are given names based on their location along the meridian on which they are found. For example, Kidney 1, abbreviated as KD 1, is the first point on the Kidney meridian.

Acupoints also have more descriptive names. Sometimes these are anatomically descriptive, such as the traditional name for Stomach 7 (ST 7), "Below the Joint," which is located below the jaw joint. Sometimes the names are more poetic, such as "Heaven's Tripod" (LI 17) and "Welcome Fragrance" (LI 20).

Traditional point names can be so memorable, it's unfortunate how secondary their use has become in many TCM (Traditional Chinese Medicine) circles, having been replaced by labels referencing their location along the meridians. It's hard to forget the "Container of Tears," a point located just below the center of the lower eyelid. Though not recommended for the lay practitioner due to its precarious and highly sensitive location, the "Container of Tears" is a far more evocative title than its complementary label, ST 1, given its function as a regulator of excessive tearing (lacrimation).

What is a Cun?

A cun (pronounced /ts'un/) is a form of measurement used in Traditional Chinese Medicine based on measurements derived from certain parts of the receiver's body.

You can use your fingers to make cun measurements for certain parts of the body, as detailed where relevant in The Points chapter. Generally speaking, 1 cun is equal to the width of the thumb at the knuckle, 1.5 cun to the width of the two forefingers, and 3 cun to the width of four fingers.

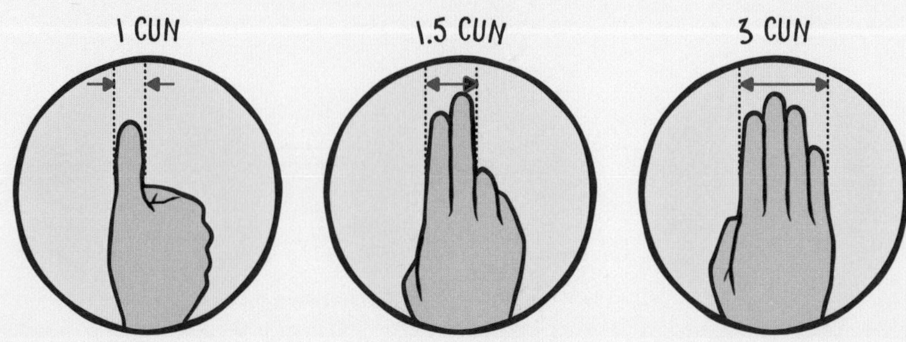

Like any evolving system of medicine, the number of acupoints changes. Currently, and depending on your source of information, there are between 300 and 600 known acupoints. This book concentrates on the 50 points labeled over the next few pages, all located on one of the 12 **principal meridians** and two **extraordinary meridians** (see page 14).

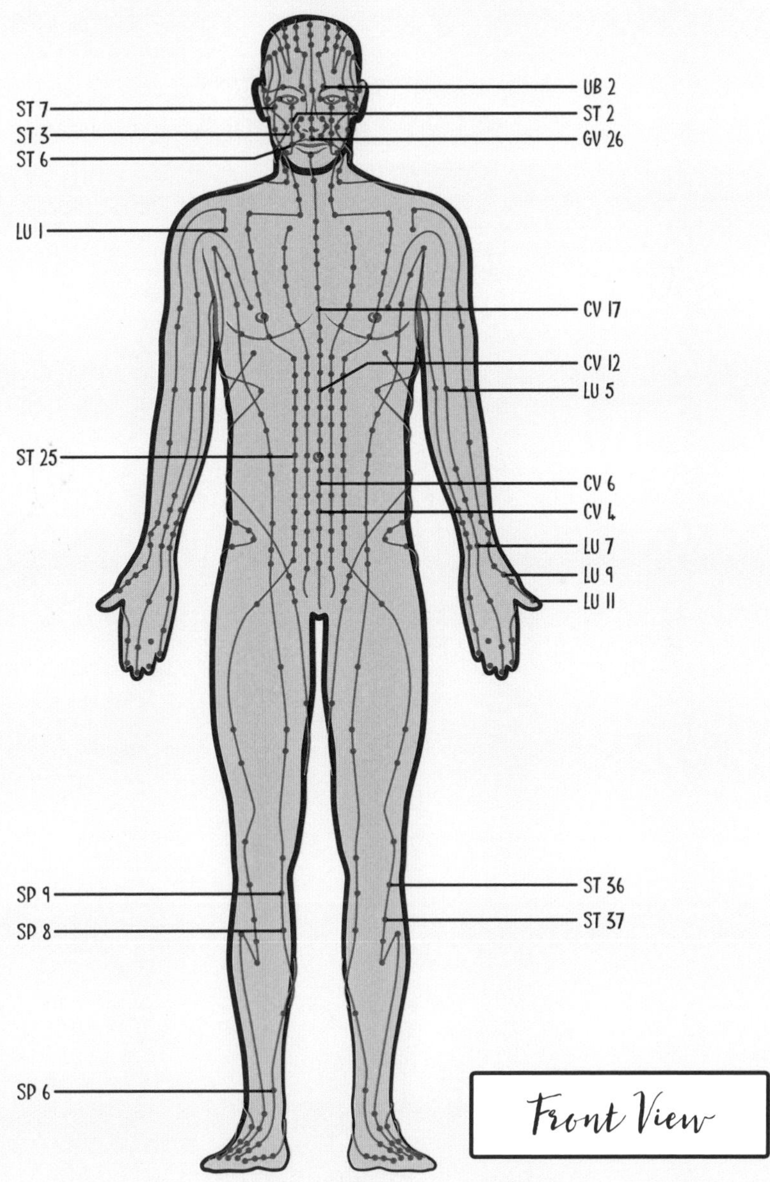

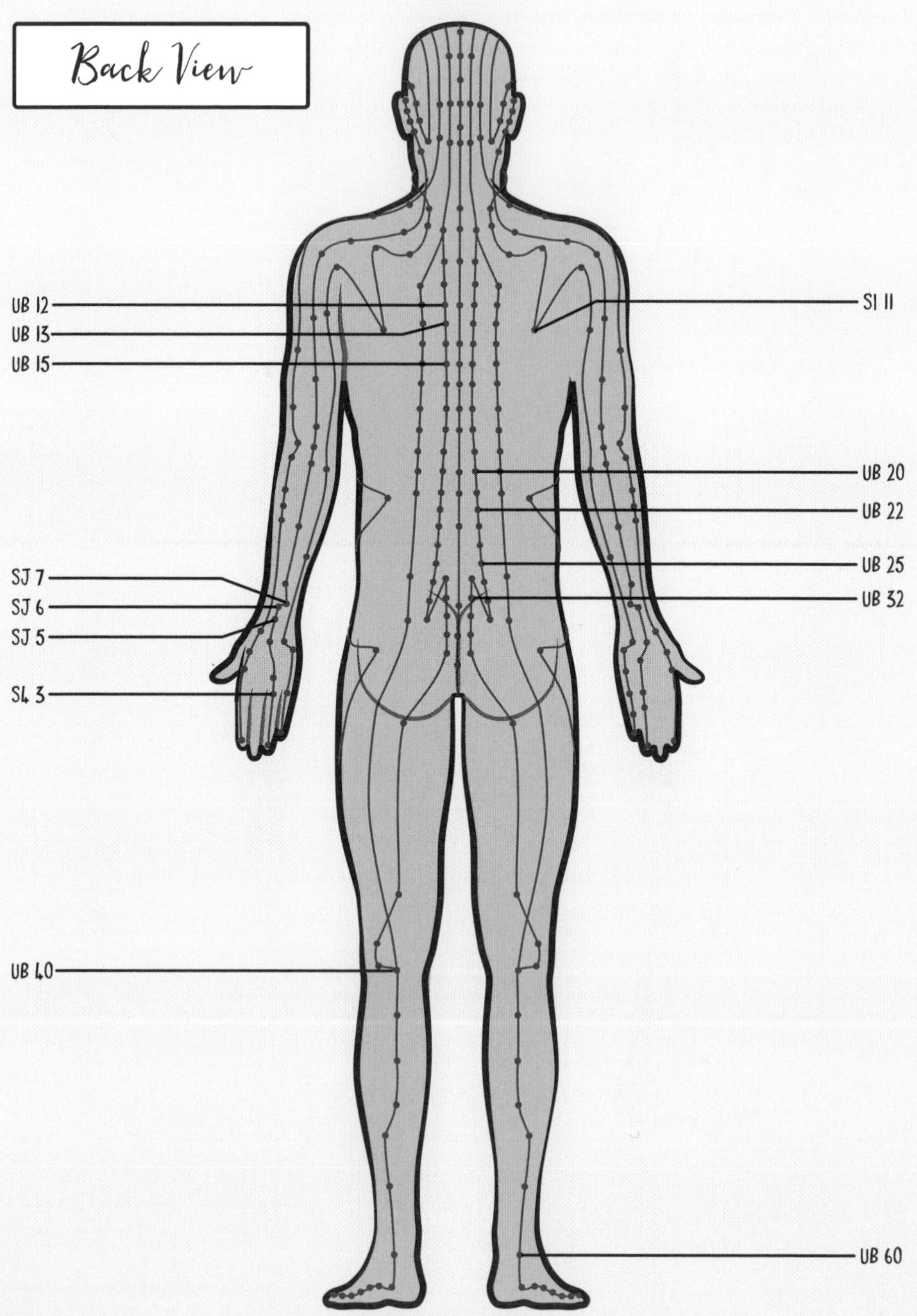
Back View
UB 12
UB 13
UB 15
SI 11
UB 20
UB 22
UB 25
UB 32
SJ 7
SJ 6
SJ 5
SI 3
UB 40
UB 60

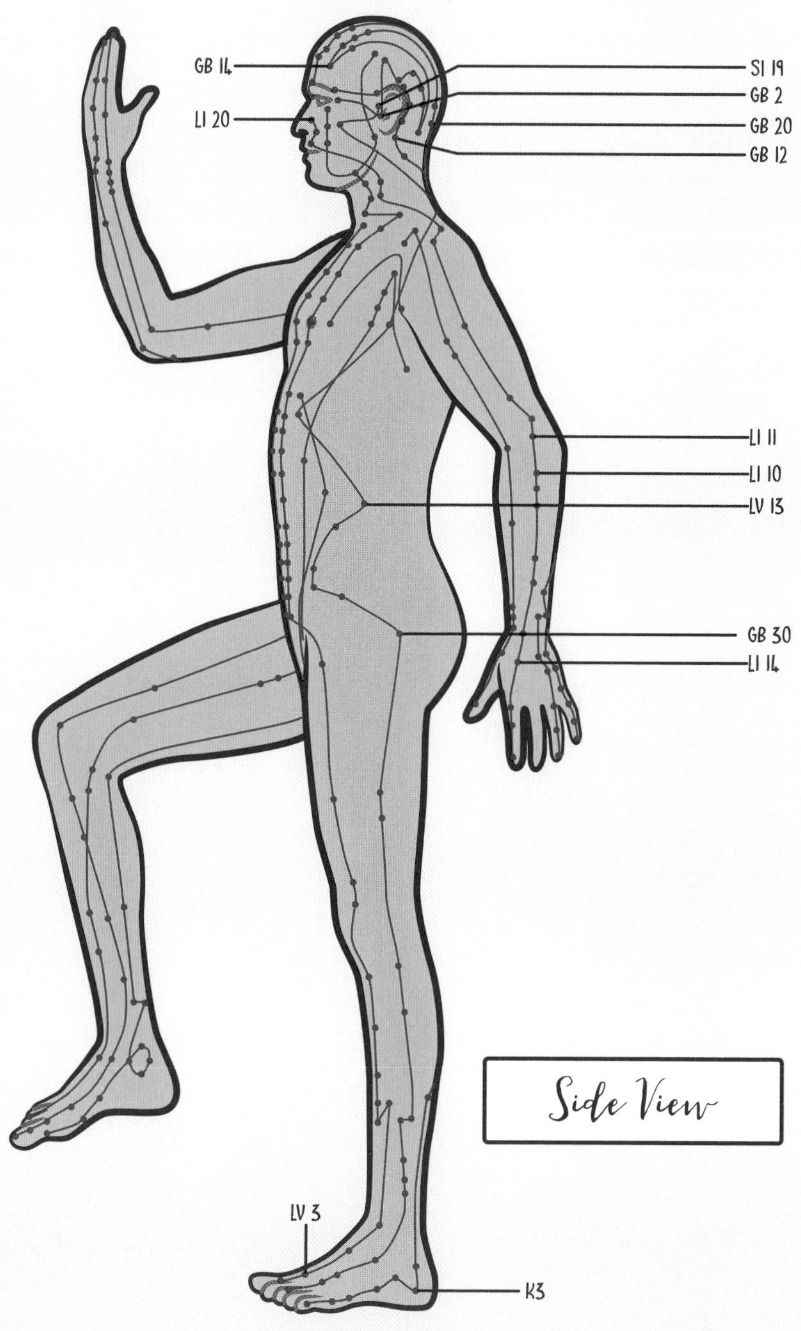
GB 14
LI 20
SI 19
GB 2
GB 20
GB 12
LI 11
LI 10
LV 13
GB 30
LI 14
Side View
LV 3
K3

USEFUL TCM CONCEPTS

Traditional Chinese Medicine is filled with enumerable poetic and evocative concepts and terms that can be confusing to those who are unaccustomed to them. Below are a handful of some of the most commonly encountered ones.

Yin/Yang

Most people have heard of the terms **Yin** and **Yang**, or may even own a piece of jewelry adorned with the Yin-Yang symbol. Although known primarily as a concept of balance, based around the idea that when dealing with opposites there's always a bit of each in the other, both Yin and Yang are distinct, yet complementary, concepts.

Yin has to do with the cool and sometimes dark aspects of our natural environment. Cold, passive, darkness, shadowy, receptive, nighttime, and shade are all associated with Yin.

Yang is all about action and heat. Warmth, sun, daytime, and movement are associated with Yang.

Six "Evils"

Traditional Chinese Medicine takes into account what it calls the six "Evils" or influences that can affect the body and mind. These are: Wind, Cold, Heat, Dryness, Dampness, and Fire (also known as Summer Heat). There are also numerous combinations to be aware of, which are far too involved for the book that you hold in your hand, such as Wind-Cold, Wind-Heat, and Damp-Heat.

WIND

Wind in Chinese Medicine is seen as the bringer of bad things, and is often considered the greatest of the "evils." Colds, flu, and most other external pathogens travel via Wind.

COLD

Cold is known for its stagnating quality where, when in excess, **qi**, **blood**, and **lymph** come to a crawl, or worse, a grinding halt in the body. Symptoms such as chills, congestion, cramping, and stiffness are all associated with Cold.

HEAT

An **excess** in Heat is dangerous to the body, primarily because of its damaging effect on the fluids. Heat dries the body out, making it susceptible to many other issues, including fever, thirst, itching, and irritability.

DRYNESS

Dryness is sometimes mistaken for Heat, in so much as the two share some similar qualities. However, Dryness is more often than not described in relation to the lungs. Symptoms of Dryness include a dry tongue, mouth and lips, a dry cough, dry stools that cause constipation, and thirst.

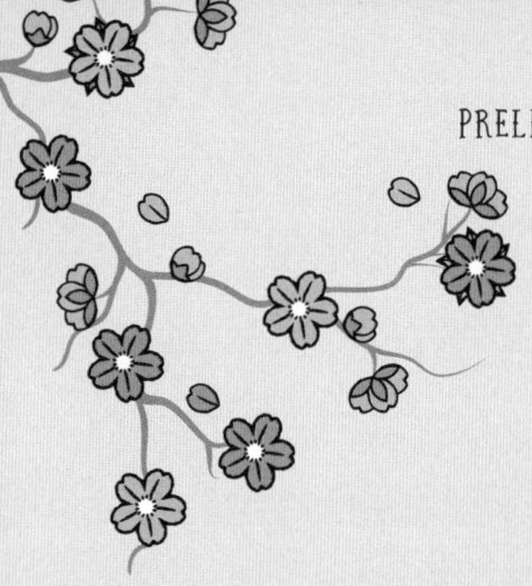

DAMPNESS

The qualities of Dampness are reflected in the word itself. Slow and sluggish, Dampness is often experienced as heaviness, greasiness, swelling, bad-smelling discharges, and mucus.

FIRE/SUMMER HEAT

Fire/Summer Heat is an external pathogen whose effects are environmental in nature. Think heatstroke and excess of perspiration with a great need for replenishing fluids, and you're on the right track.

Excess and Deficiency

TCM also considers whether a condition may be in excess or in a state of deficiency, which describe the lack or proliferation of substances, "evils," and qualities in the body.

EXCESS

Excess is associated with fullness; however, more than that, it has to do with resistance and pushing back. Consider an injury you may have had that made you recoil when touched. That is a sign of excess.

DEFICIENCY

Deficiency has to do with emptiness, but, like excess, takes it one step further. Think back to a massage you may have had when, although a spot may have been tender, you could not take enough pressure. So much so that you wished the therapist would press right through you into the table. That is a sign of deficiency.

Organs

The concept of organs in Chinese medicine is sometimes confusing to outsiders. While there are certainly similarities between the Western and Chinese anatomical understanding of what the organs are, and the functions they peform, TCM also considers the energetic, as well as metaphoric, significance of an organ.

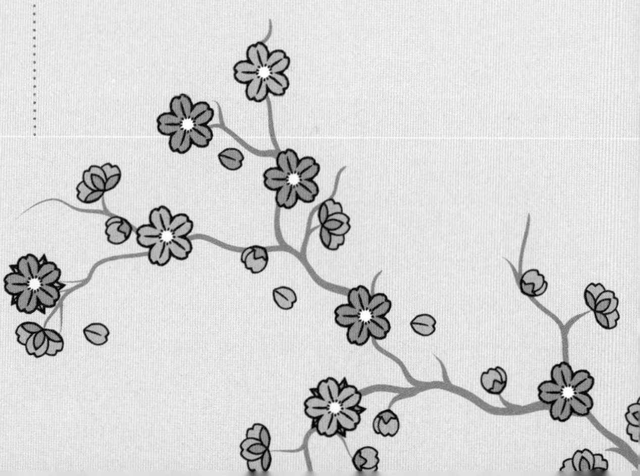

2 GUIDELINES & APPROACHES

Each of us has a unique part to play in the healing of the world.

MARIANNE WILLIAMSON

BASIC ANATOMY OF THE HAND

Before there were needles for acupuncture, glass globes for cupping therapy, and even fire for lighting moxa, we had our **hands**. To write about the intelligence of our hands would take an entire book. Suffice it to say, we mammals have been using our hands for complex activities, including **healing**, since we decided to turn in our flippers.

Think back to pictures you've seen of gorillas grooming one another in the forest. While this activity is certainly a form of bonding between mammals, it is also a type of basic medicine, especially when you consider how critters that crawl over the skin might irritate the tissue, or worse, impart diseases to the body.

Healing with our hands can be seen as a complex extension of that very fundamental grooming practice. Only, rather than removing external irritants, we are helping to **regulate internal systems**, both physical and energetic.

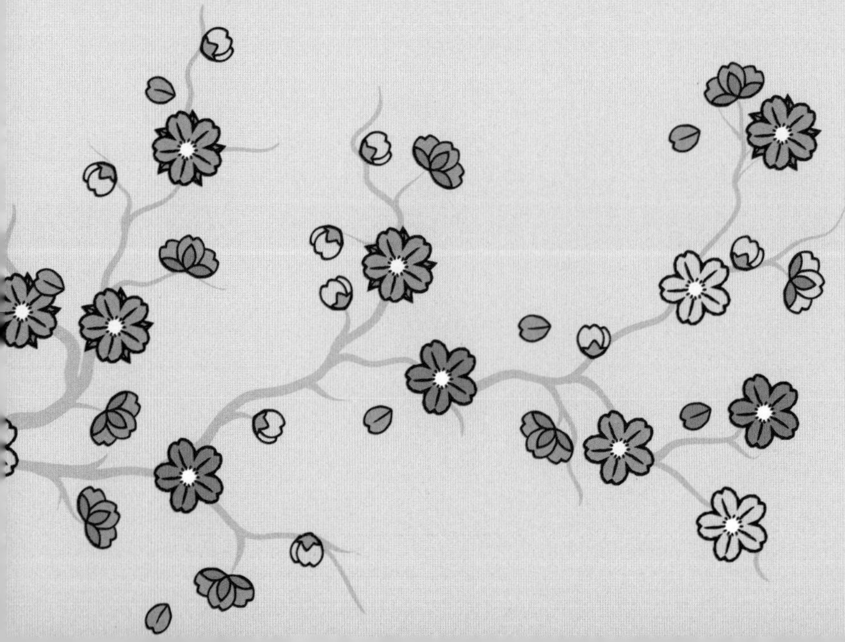

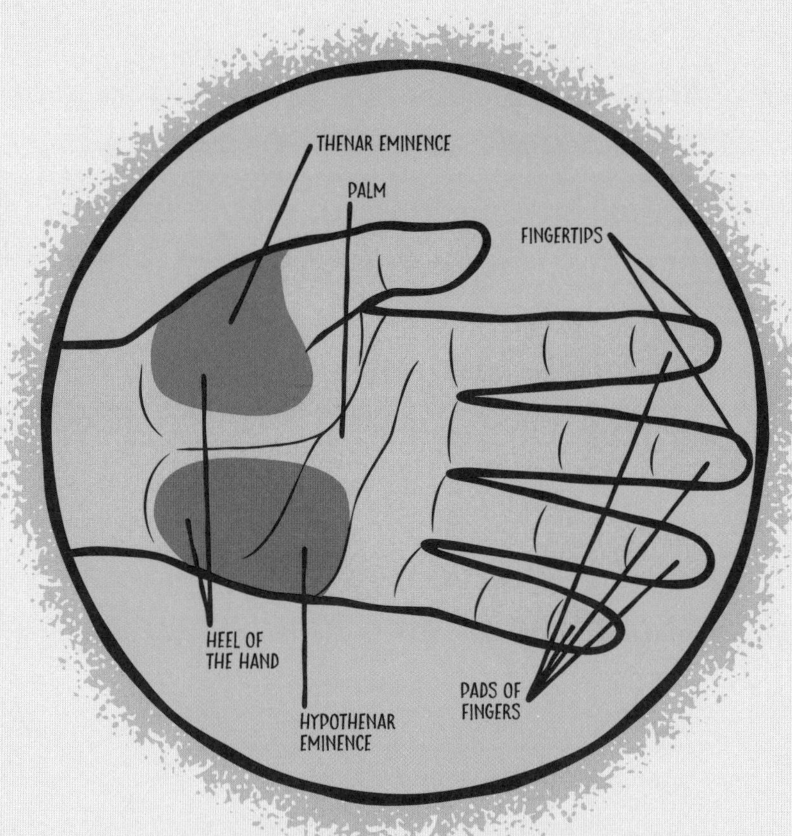

Acupressure is administered primarily with the use of our hands. Depending on the effect we would like to achieve, practitioners will use different parts of the hand. For example, to offer a gentle and calming stimulation, a practitioner may use the thenar eminence. For more acute work that may give a client a feeling of "good pain" (pain that is not jarring or abrasive, but therapeutic in nature), the practitioner may use the tips of the fingers.

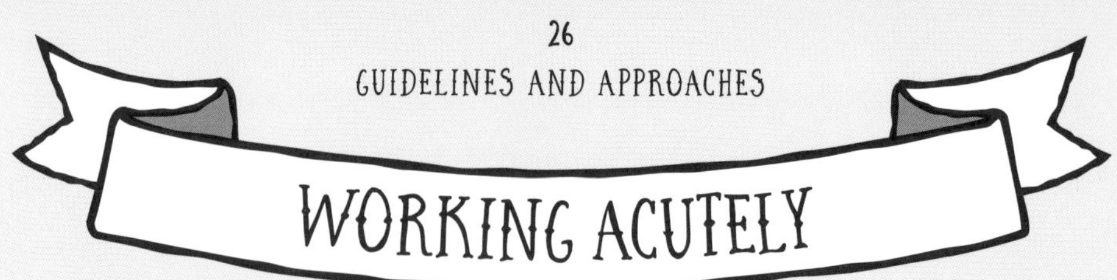

WORKING ACUTELY

When working an acupoint we often need to choose between working **acutely**—with fingers, thumbs, and elbows—or **generally**—with palms, loose fists, or forearms. Decisions on what "tool" to use depends on what we want to achieve, as well as how the person is receiving the work. In most instances, you will find yourself working on very specific **point locations** on the body.

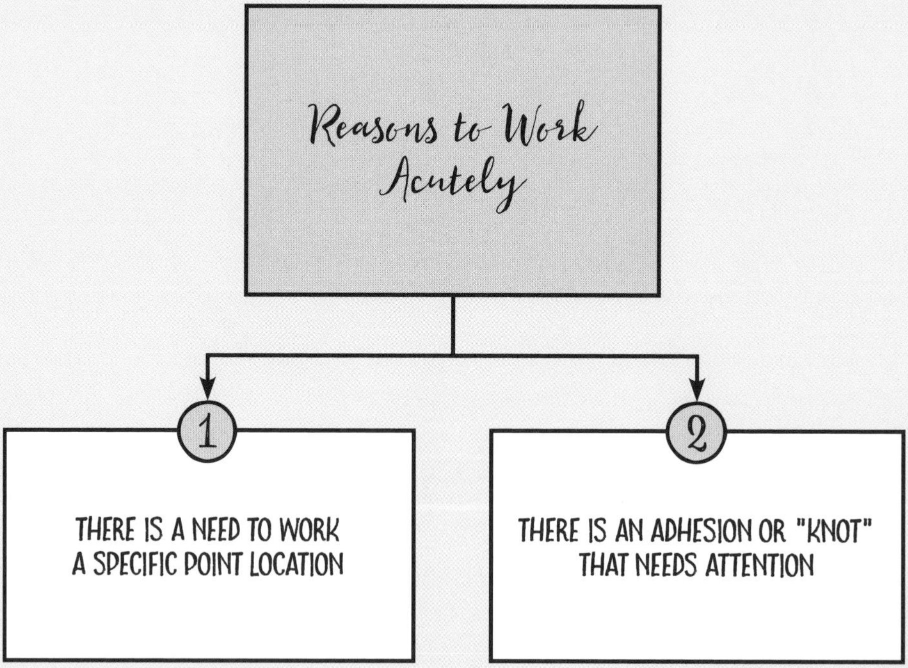

Reasons to Work Acutely

1. THERE IS A NEED TO WORK A SPECIFIC POINT LOCATION
2. THERE IS AN ADHESION OR "KNOT" THAT NEEDS ATTENTION

WORKING ACUTELY LOOKS LIKE THIS

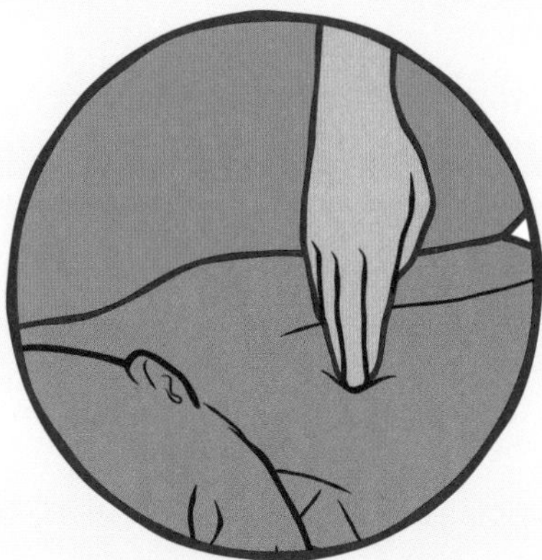

Bring both the ring and index fingers behind the middle finger, which is the primary point of contact. The other two fingers will be used mainly for support.

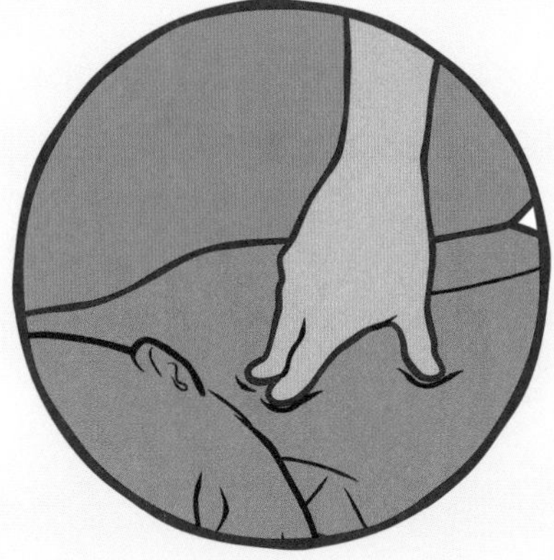

Though it seems obvious to use them, thumbs are not as strong as one would think. Be gentle when beginning to use your thumbs for acupressure work. Line up the thumbs with the wrist, as shown above, and they will last you a lifetime.

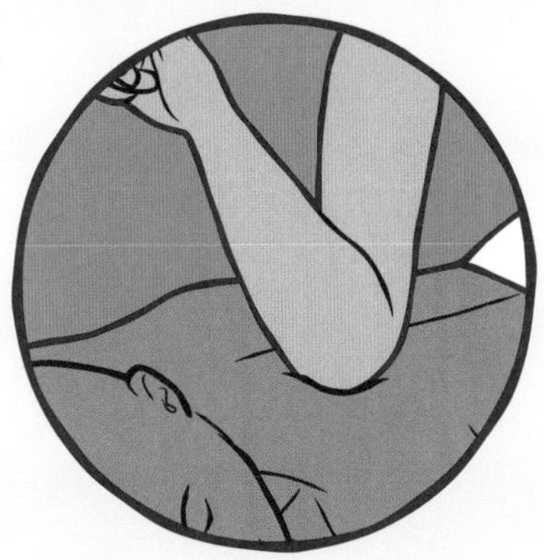

Elbows are great for points that just won't release. They are also heavy and powerful. Always check in with the receiver regarding pressure: start softly, and work only as deep as the receiver wants.

WORKING GENERALLY

Working **generally** means to work over a slightly **broader area** or region of the body than when working acutely (see pages 26–27).

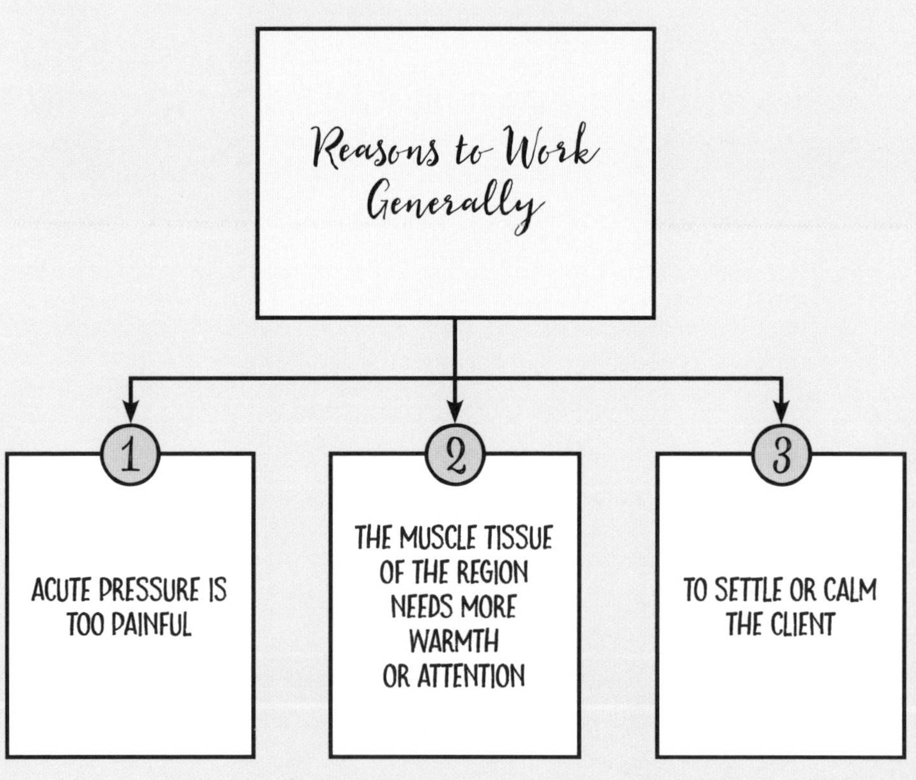

Reasons to Work Generally
1
ACUTE PRESSURE IS TOO PAINFUL
2
THE MUSCLE TISSUE OF THE REGION NEEDS MORE WARMTH OR ATTENTION
3
TO SETTLE OR CALM THE CLIENT

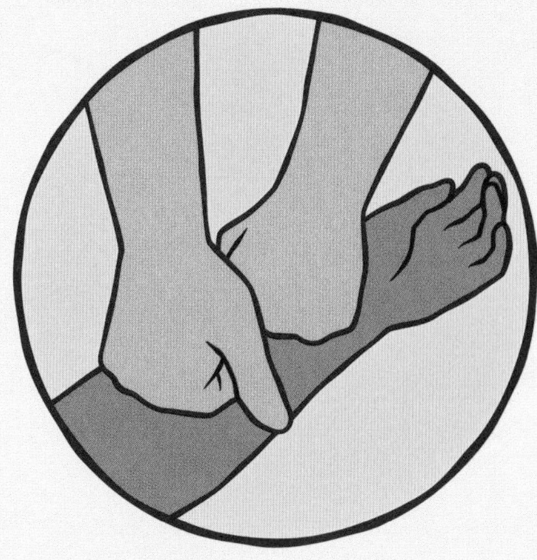

Loose fists can provide deeper pressure than some of the other general techniques, but still have the effect of being broad and warming.

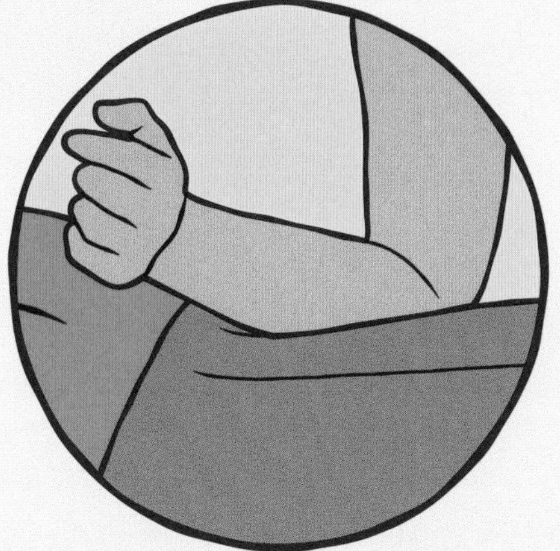

Forearms are a great middle ground between acute elbow work and loose fists. The method is broad in feeling, but can be deep in pressure if needed.

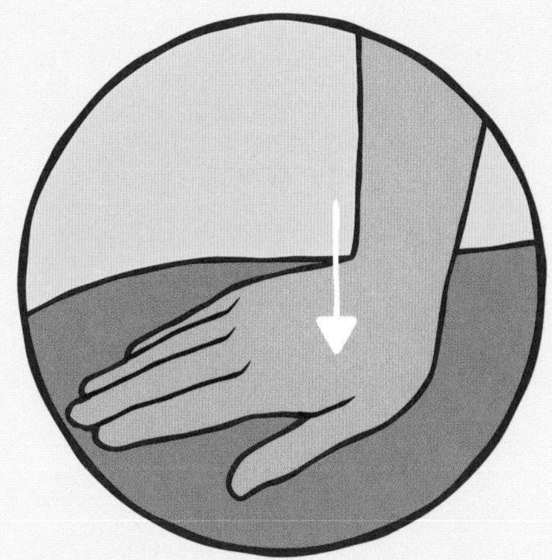

An open palm offers a broad and warming approach to acupressure work. While far less acute than other approaches, an open palm can have a very nurturing quality.

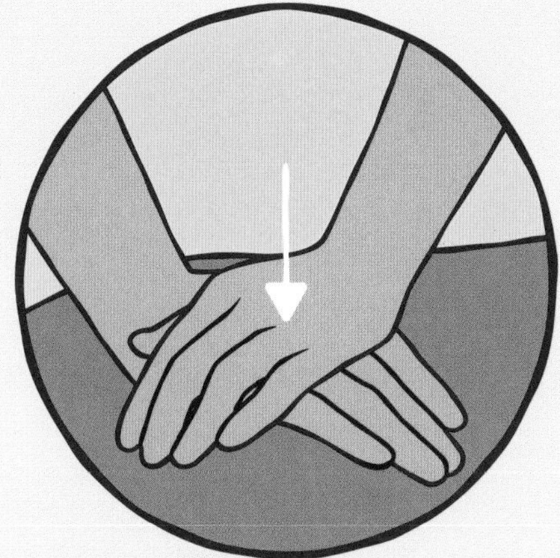

Place one palm over the other to apply more pressure and to support your own wrists and hands.

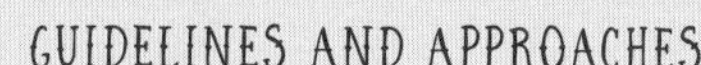

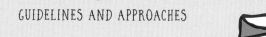

GUIDELINES FOR APPLYING PRESSURE

As pleasurable as it can be, there is much more to acupressure than pressing a tender point on the body. While there is certainly some truth to this common misconception—since tender points on the body can at times be alleviated with direct pressure—to have a truly effective treatment, one should become familiar with some guidelines for approaching points.

1

Locate the Point

POINT LOCATION IS A SKILL ALL ITS OWN. USING BOTH ANATOMICAL LANDMARKS, AS WELL AS MEASUREMENTS BASED ON PARTS OF THE CLIENT'S BODY (SEE PAGES 16-19), WITH PRACTICE YOU WILL GAIN A SENSITIVITY THAT WILL ALLOW YOU TO FIND AND FEEL ACUPOINTS WITH EASE.

2

Warm the Area

IN CHINESE MASSAGE, KNEADING AN AREA OF THE BODY IN A CIRCULAR FASHION WITH THE THUMB, FINGERTIPS, OR FOREARM IS A TECHNIQUE KNOWN AS "ROU FA" OR ROUND RUBBING. BEFORE APPLYING PRESSURE DIRECTLY TO ANY ACUPOINT, WARM THE AREA WITH THIS SIMPLE TECHNIQUE WHILE APPLYING ENOUGH PRESSURE TO GENERATE HEAT AND SOFTEN THE MUSCLE TISSUE. SOFTENING THE TISSUE BEFORE APPLYING MORE STATIC PRESSURE WILL NOT ONLY MAKE THE POINT MORE ACCESSIBLE, BUT ALSO GIVE YOU A BETTER SENSE OF HOW THE POINT RELATES AND INTERACTS WITH THE SURROUNDING ANATOMY.

3

Add Pressure

ONCE YOU HAVE LOCATED THE POINT, AND BROUGHT WARMTH TO THE AREA, YOU ARE READY TO APPLY PRESSURE. TO WORK ACUTELY, USE EITHER THE PADS OF YOUR THUMBS OR BRING THE TIPS OF YOUR INDEX, MIDDLE, AND RING FINGERS TO A POINT AND PRESS INTO THE AREA YOU ARE WORKING.

4

Slow Circular Motions

TO INCREASE THE EFFICACY OF YOUR TECHNIQUE YOU MAY WANT TO MAKE SLOW CIRCULAR MOTIONS, WHICH YOU CAN INCREASE IN PRESSURE AS MUCH AS THE RECEIVER IS ABLE TO ACCEPT. MAKING CIRCULAR MOTIONS WILL ALSO HELP TO MAINTAIN WARMTH IN THE AREA.

5

Duration of Hold

THERE IS NO SET RULE ON HOW LONG A POINT CAN AND SHOULD BE HELD. I HAVE HELD A POINT FOR AS LITTLE AS THREE SECONDS AND AS LONG AS THREE MINUTES. ACUPUNCTURISTS WILL SOMETIMES ADHESE SMALL BLACK SEEDS TO POINTS THAT WILL MAINTAIN PRESSURE ON A POINT FOR HOURS AT A TIME. SO, REALLY, THE SKY IS THE LIMIT. HOWEVER, TYPICALLY, 90 SECONDS TO 3 MINUTES IS CONSIDERED ADEQUATE.

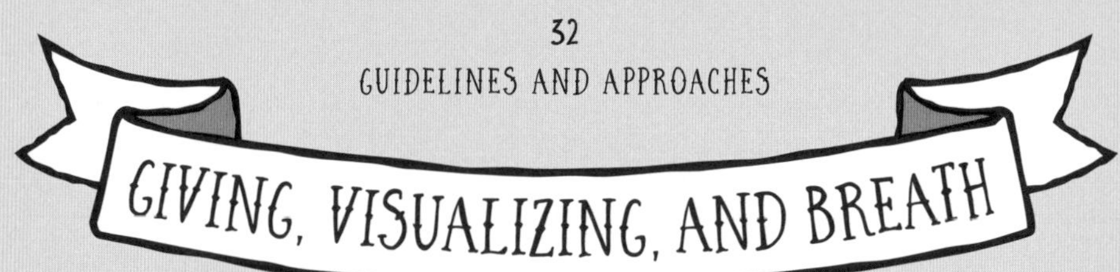

GIVING, VISUALIZING, AND BREATH

Giving an acupressure treatment involves more than pressing points on the body. While the pressure itself is very important, using our abilities to visualize the work **we hope to accomplish**, as well as using our breath to direct both the pressure and the visualization, can mean the difference between a treatment that works and one that falls flat.

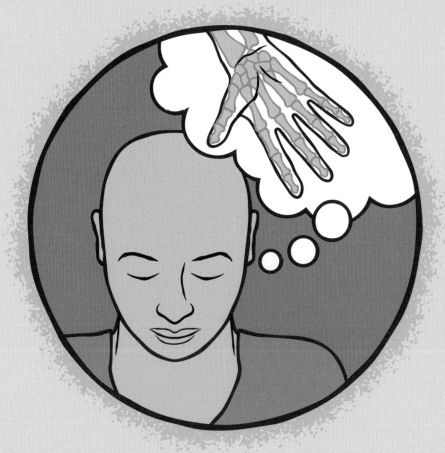

Visualization involves seeing in your mind both the anatomical structures you are working on, as well as the energetic pool of **qi** you want to **manipulate**.

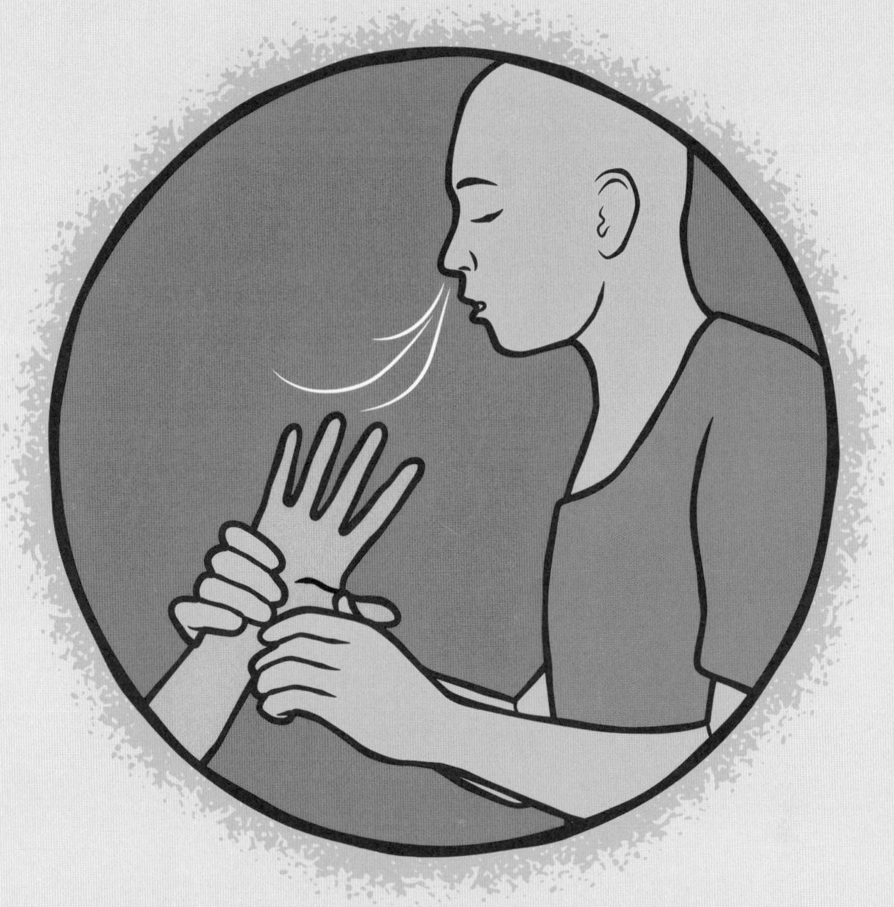

Matching your breath to the work you are performing is essential. As a rule of thumb, you want to use **exhales** when **applying** pressure, and **inhales** when **releasing** pressure.

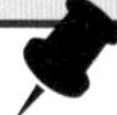

NOTE

Always try to breathe through your nose, rather than your mouth. Nothing kills the vibe of a session more than a practitioner breathing heavily out of their mouth. Breathing through the nose is not only healthier (the nose filters the air we breathe), but is also more efficient for the body, because it warms the outside air before it enters the lungs.

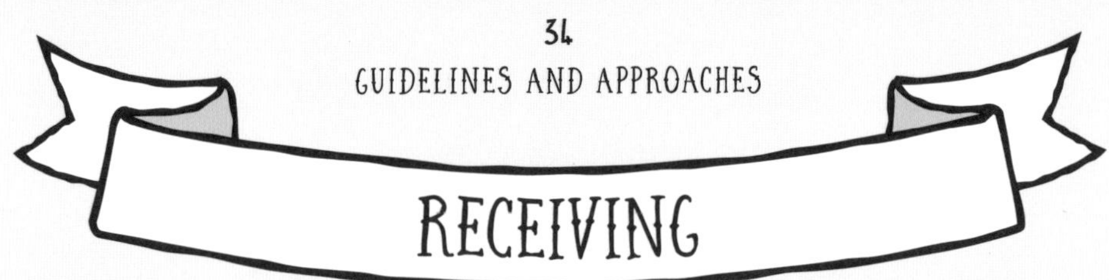

RECEIVING

Acupressure treatments are known for their extremely **calming** effects on the receiver. However, there are many ways to come to that place of serenity! Throughout a treatment, whether given by yourself or by a practitioner, you may find yourself experiencing a number of different sensations depending on the state of the points being worked on.

Warmth

Often when a point is pressed you will feel a **warming sensation**. We tend to read this sensation as a result of increased activity in the region, whether it be **qi**, blood, or, as is most often the case, both!

Cooling

Sometimes you may feel a **cooling sensation** around the point being worked. In these cases, this may be to do with the blood being momentarily drained from the area. Blood briefly moving out of an area of muscle tissue makes room for new blood to flood back in when the pressure is released. This is perfectly normal, and so long as there is no tingling associated with this coolness, it is perfectly healthy. If, however, there is a tingling sensation, slowly release the pressure, and let the sensation dissipate.

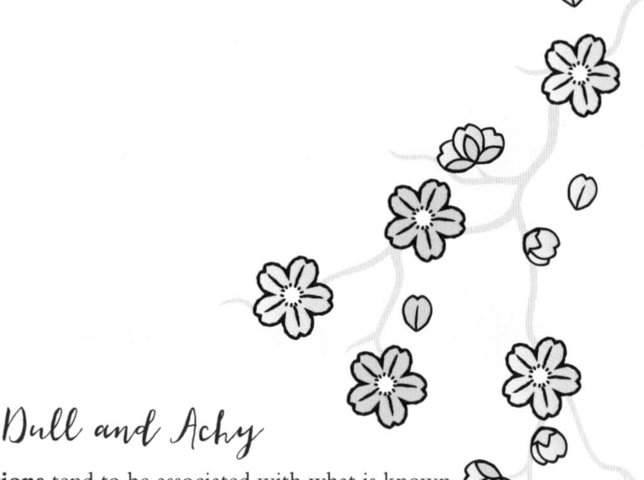

Dull and Achy

Dull, **achy sensations** tend to be associated with what is known as **deficiency** in Chinese Medicine (see page 21). This is the sensation that most people describe as “good pain” or “yummy pain.” It is the type of slightly tender feelings in the muscle that means your body is saying, “Yes, please press this area more!”

Sharp and Shooting

The only truly contraindicated sensation (in addition to tingling) that we want to avoid is the feeling of **sharp shooting pain**. This is what we would refer to as “bad pain,” and is often ascribed to the Chinese Medicine concept of **excess** (see page 21). While excess conditions are totally within the realm of workable conditions, Excess that is attributed to sharp shooting pain is to be avoided. If you come across a point that yields a sharp shooting pain when pressed, let up on the pressure and wait for the sensation to die down.

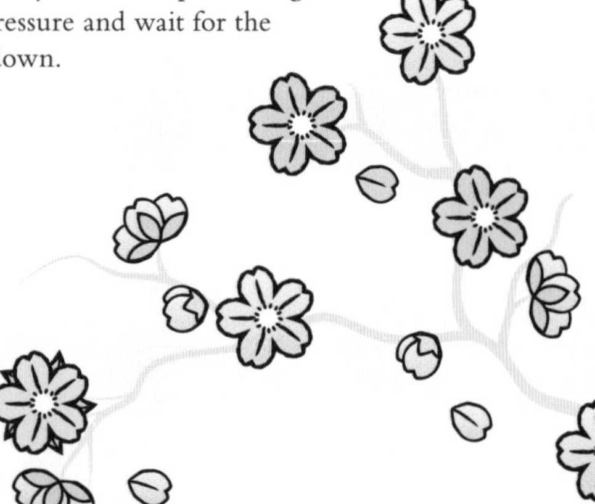

3 THE POINTS

Too often we underestimate the power of a touch, a smile, a kind word, a listening ear, an honest compliment, or the smallest act of caring, all of which have the potential to turn a life around.

LEO F. BUSCAGLIA

LU 1: CENTRAL PALACE

In the depression between the outside of the chest and the arm, 6 cun from the center line, at the level of the first intercostal space.

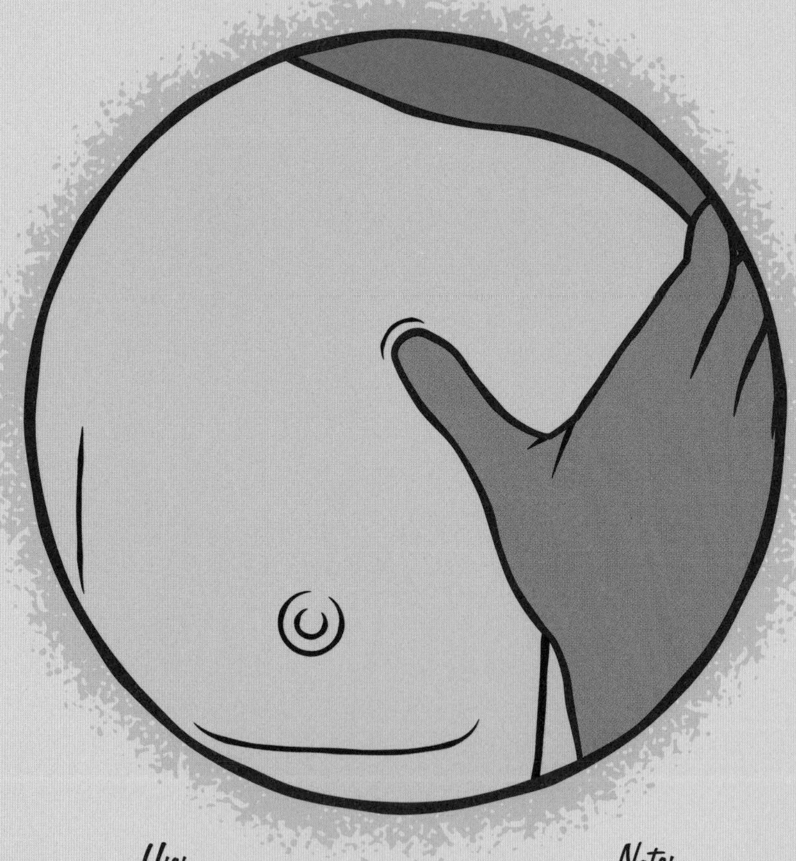

Uses

Can be used for many respiratory issues, including coughing and wheezing, as well as for chest and shoulder pain. Helps disperse heat and break up phlegm in the chest.

Notes

Often tender for those who suffer from asthma, LU 1 is especially useful when helping people increase their lung capacity. Massaging the point while taking deep breaths can be of great service to shallow breathers.

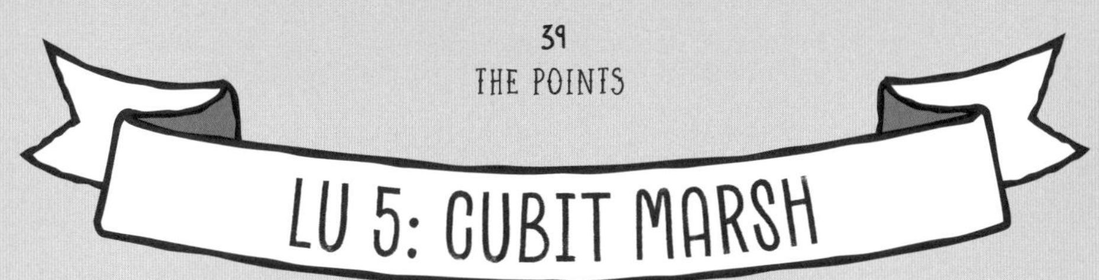

LU 5: CUBIT MARSH

Located at the crease in the elbow on the radial side of the biceps brachii tendon.

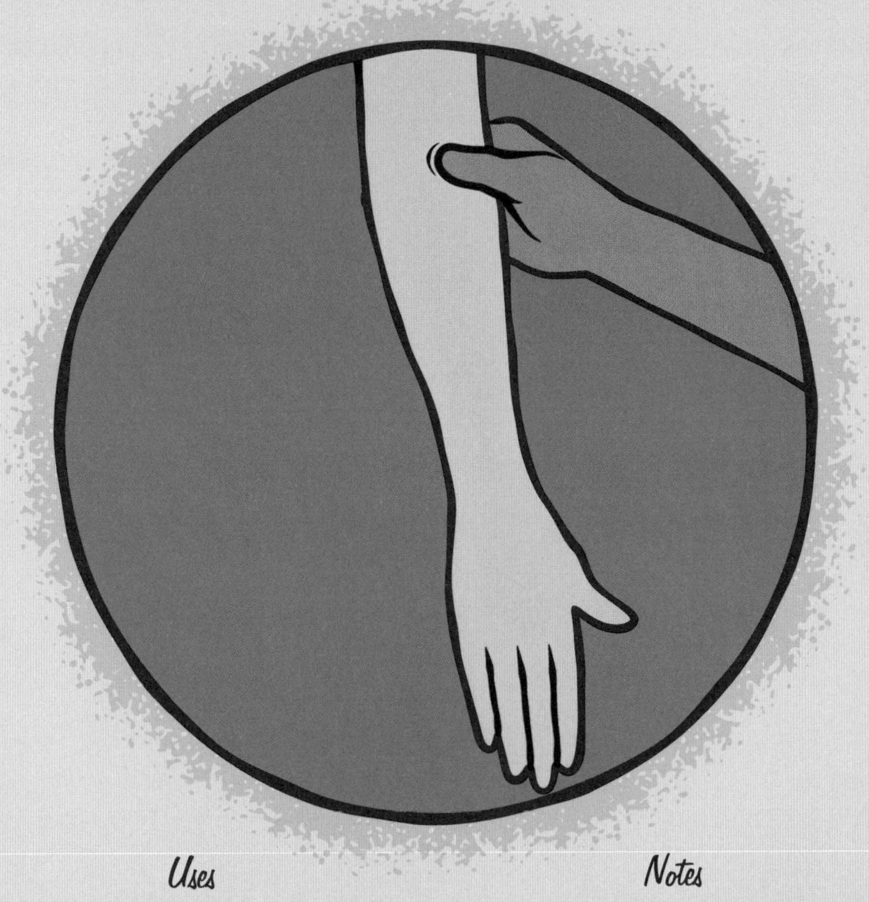

Uses

Commonly used for local elbow issues, as well as coughing, chest congestion, and sore throat.

Notes

Some consider LU 5 to be the arm equivalent to UB 40 (see page 68), and use this point for lower back pain.

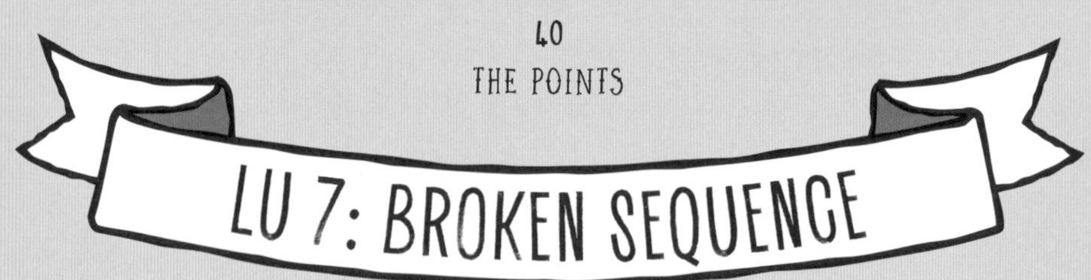

LU 7: BROKEN SEQUENCE

Located on the radial side of the lower forearm, 1.5 cun above the crease of the wrist.

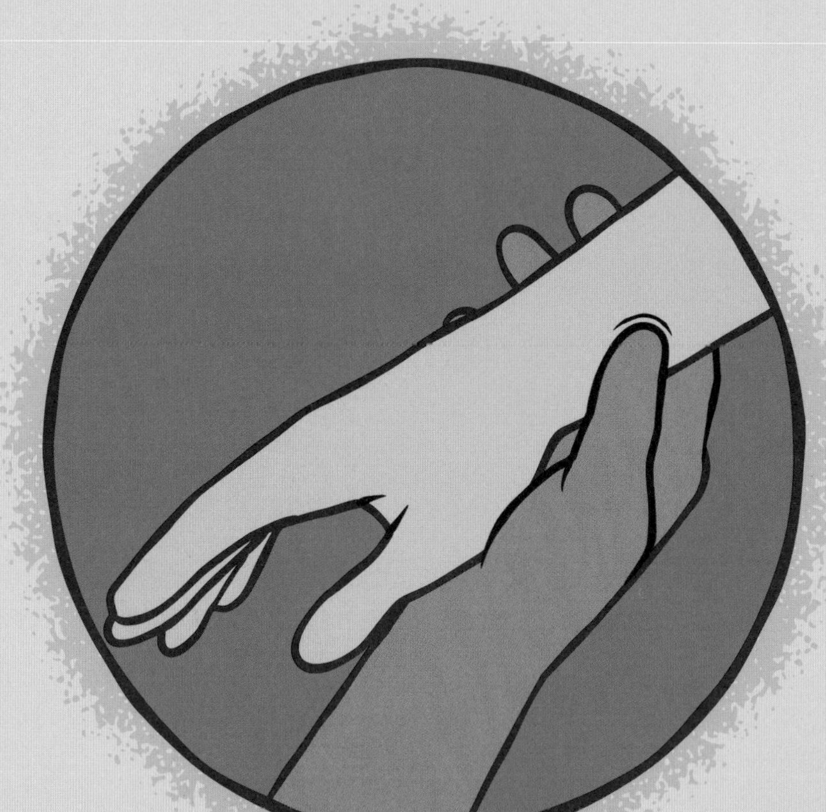

Uses

Commonly used for head and neck issues related to migraines, headaches, stiffness in the neck, facial paralysis, toothache, sore throat, cough, asthma, and general nasal problems.

Notes

LU 7 is considered useful for releasing Wind-Cold and Wind-Heat (see page 20).

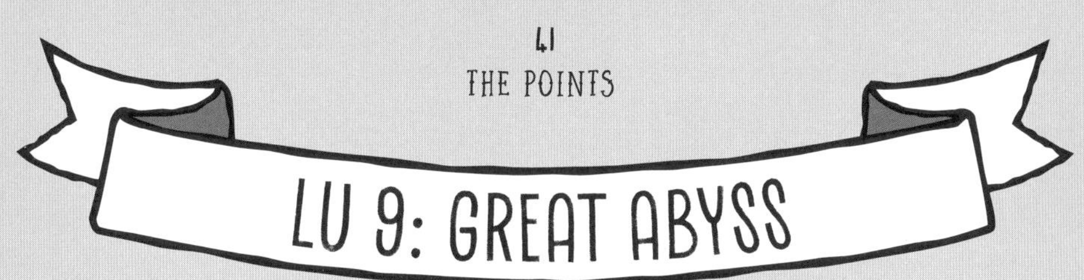

LU 9: GREAT ABYSS

Located on the thumb side of the crease of the wrist, where you can feel the radial artery pulsating.

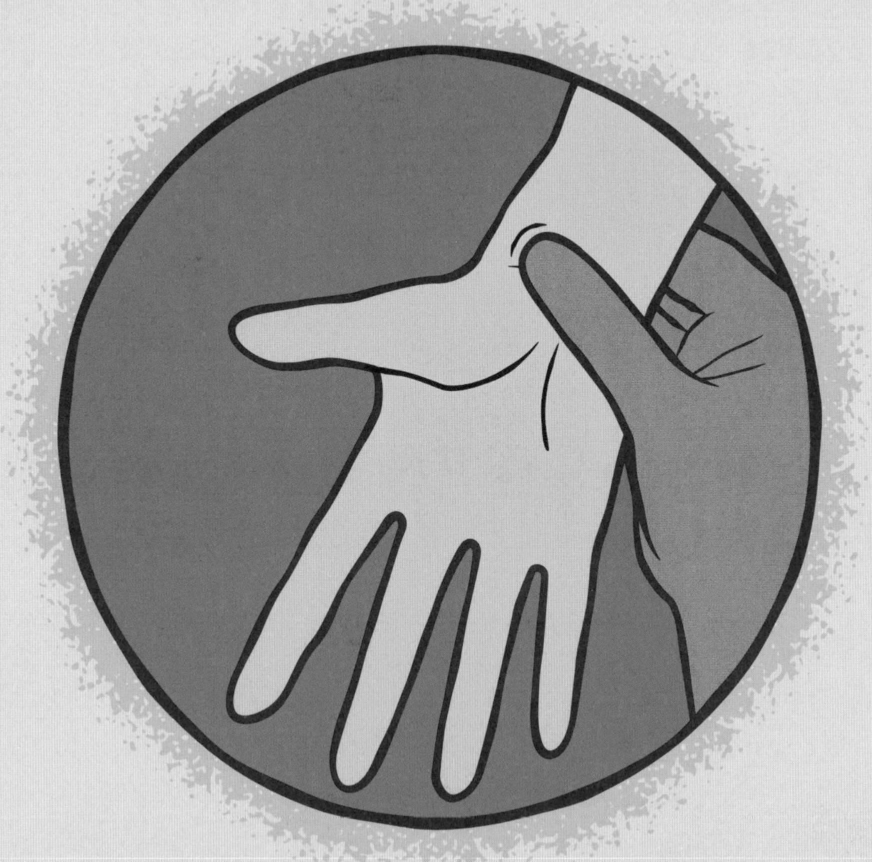

Uses

Often used for phlegmy coughs, asthma, headache, pain and weakness of the lower extremities, and wrist pain.

Notes

LU 9 is known as a great point for enhancing lung qi.

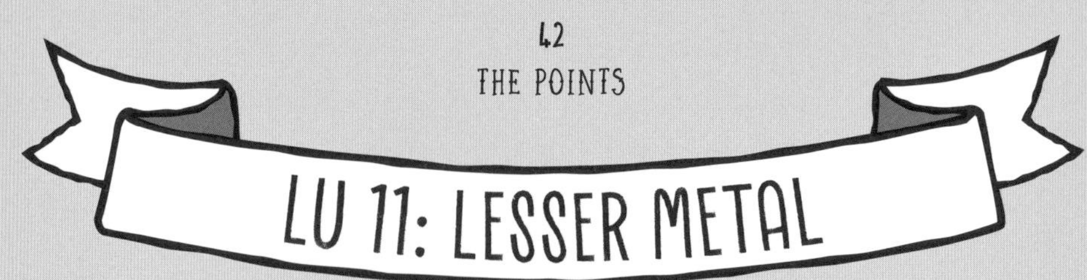

LU 11: LESSER METAL

Located at the upper outside border of the thumbnail.

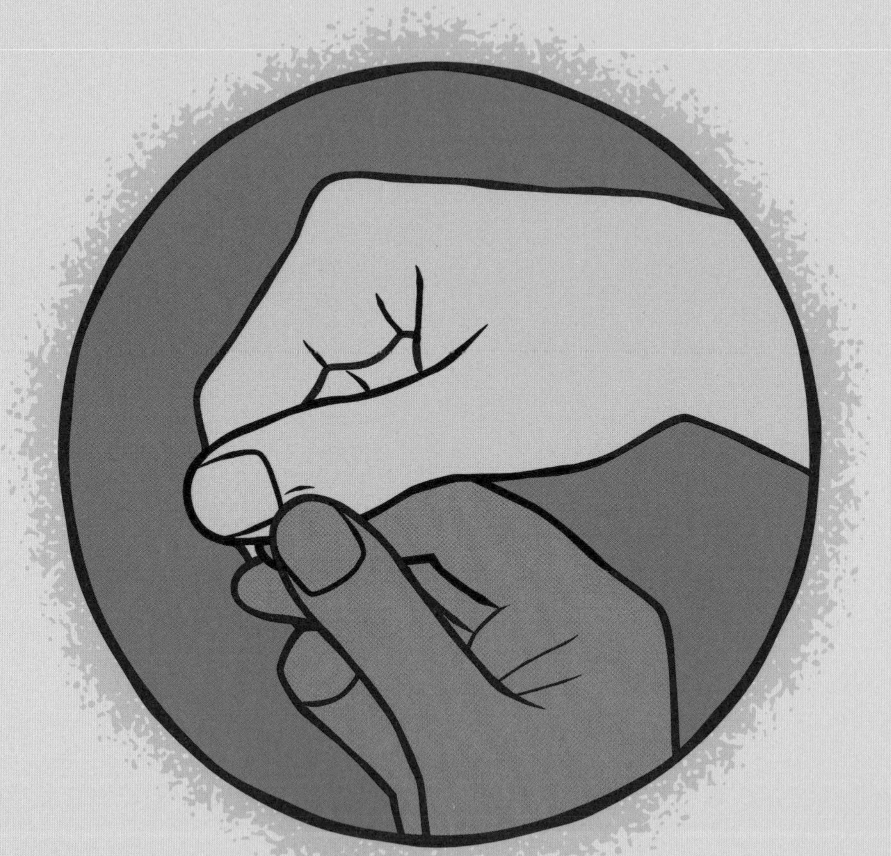

Uses

Commonly used for sore throats, coughing, fever, coma, and even manic disorders.

Notes

LU 11 is known as a Jing-Well point. Jing-Well points are areas on the meridians where the qi is said to bubble up close to the surface. These points are commonly used for reviving consciousness.

LI 4: JOINING VALLEY

On the back of the hand, in the "web" between the thumb and index finger.

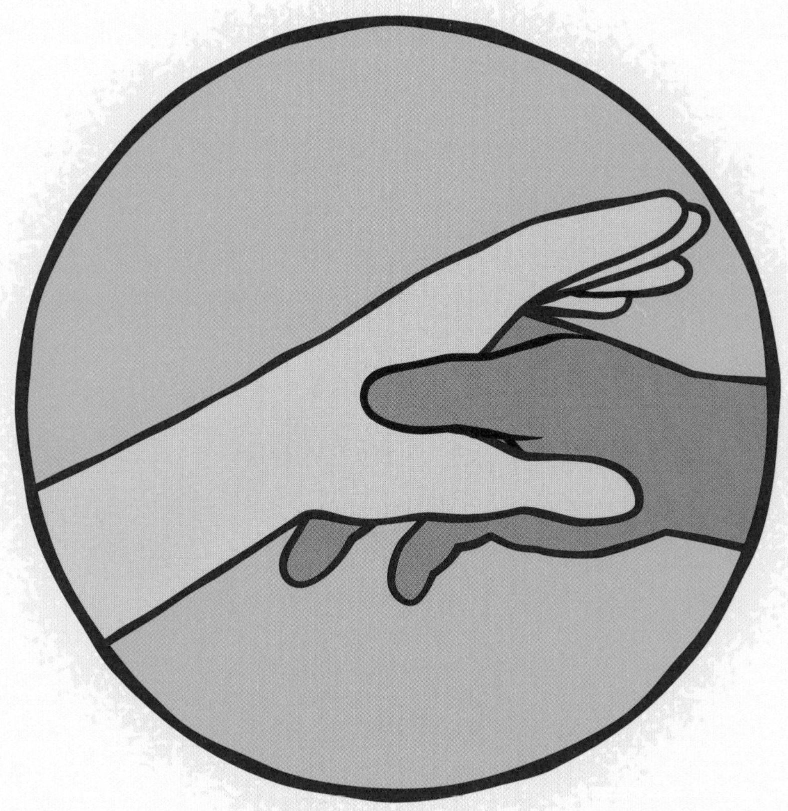

Uses

Can be used for issues relating to the head and face, uterine and gastric pain, and for strongly moving qi and blood.

Notes

One of the most well-known points, LI 4 may be used for any pain in the body, and is particularly noted for its help in relieving nausea. **Not to be used during pregnancy.**

LI 10: ARM THREE MILES

With the forearm bent, in line with the thumb, 2 cun below the crease in the elbow.

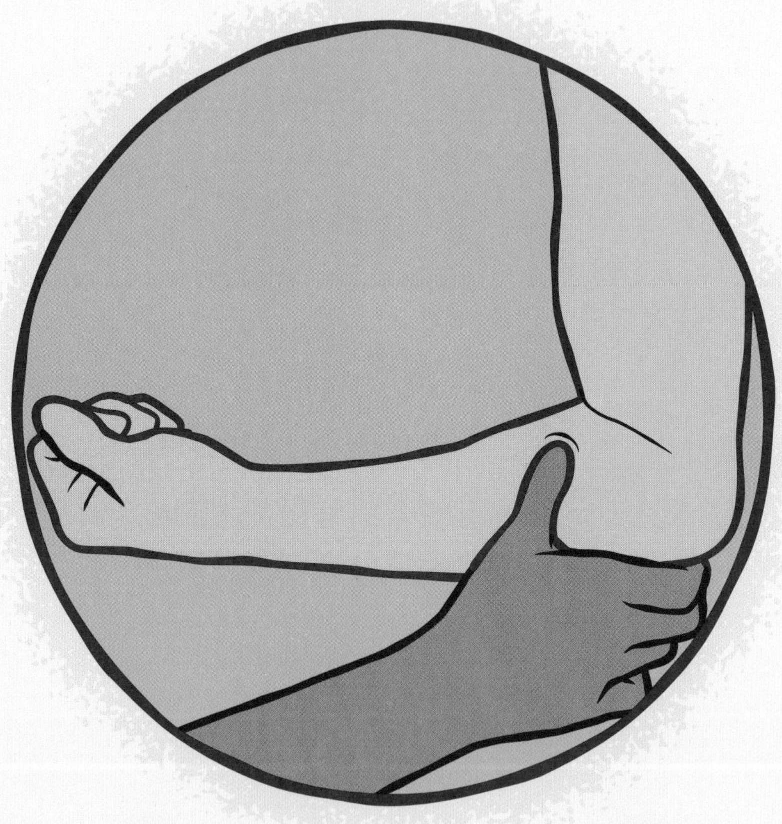

Uses

General aches and pains around the elbow, wrist, and shoulders; abdominal pain.

Notes

For issues with the arm, LI 10 can be used with similar points in the vicinity.

LI 11: POOL AT THE BEND

With arm bent across the front of the body, the point is located at the outside edge of the elbow crease.

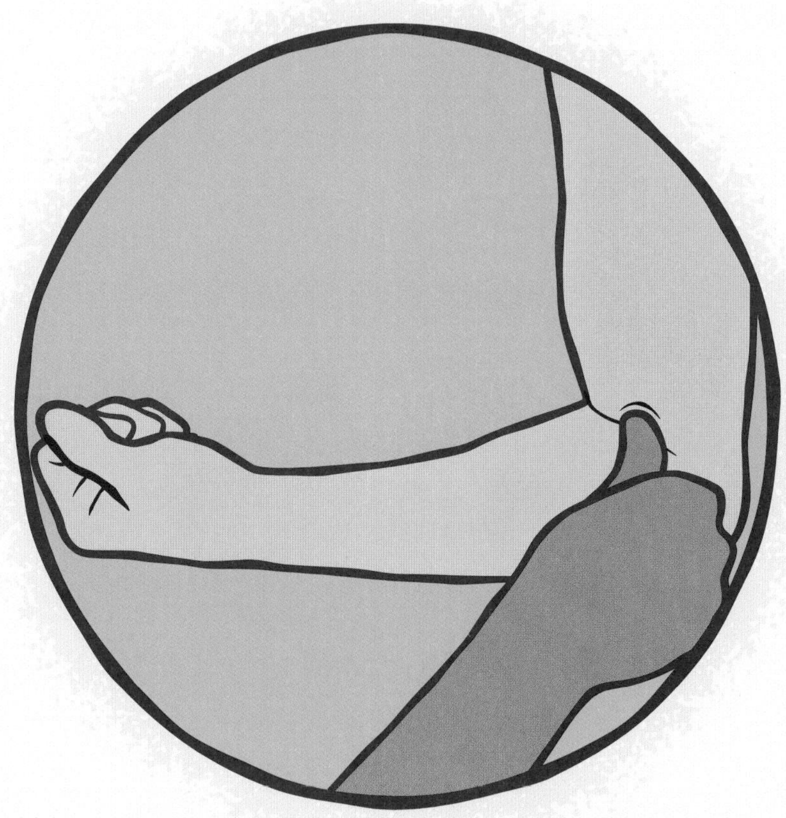

Uses

Due to its reputation as a cooling point, LI 11 helps with reduction of high fevers, heatstroke, heat-induced headaches, and heat issues related to menopause. Also used for pain around the elbow.

Notes

Qi is said to collect at this point, so using it can help with rebellious qi (burping, indigestion) and diarrhea.

LI 20: WELCOME FRAGRANCE

At the base of the nose where the "smile lines" meet the outer lower edge of the nostrils.

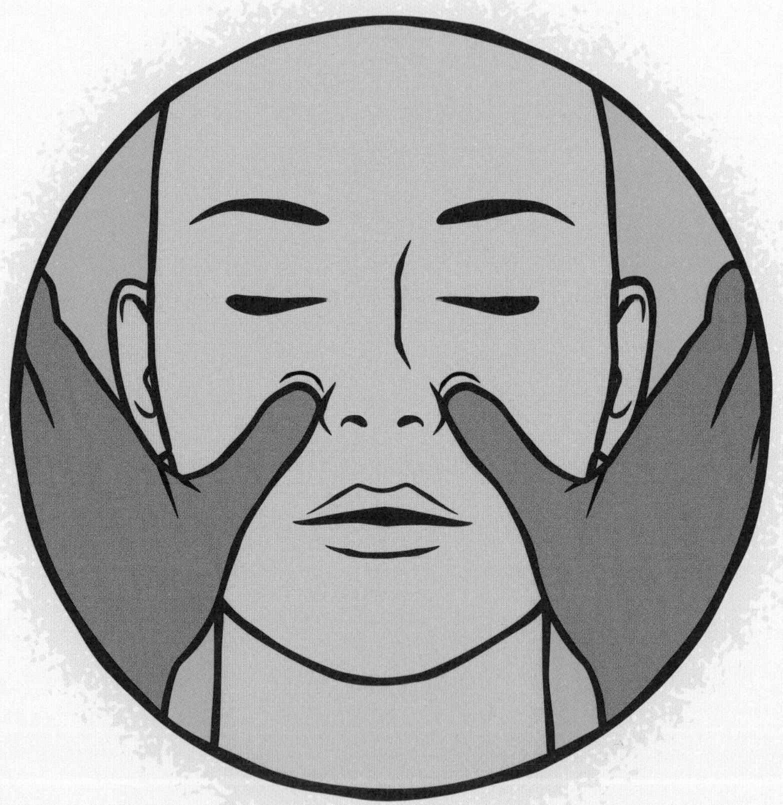

Uses

Nasal congestion, loss of smell or taste, and any nasal or sinus-related issues.

Notes

To relieve a stuffy nose, or to increase air intake, press into the point while pulling the nostrils away from one another. This is especially useful for dealing with anxiety when there is an accompanying sensation of constriction in the nasal passages.

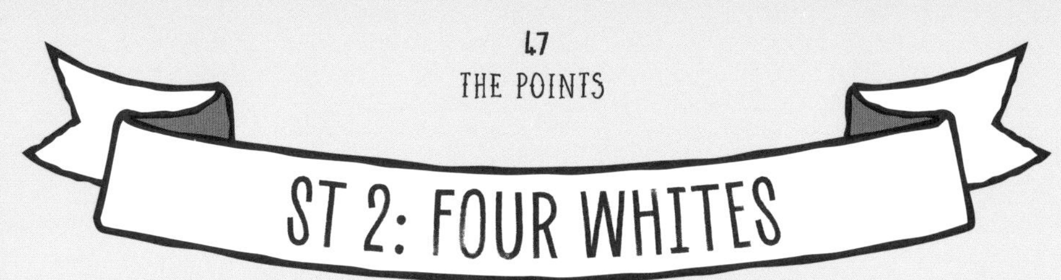

ST 2: FOUR WHITES

Located in a depression roughly 2 cun below the pupil.

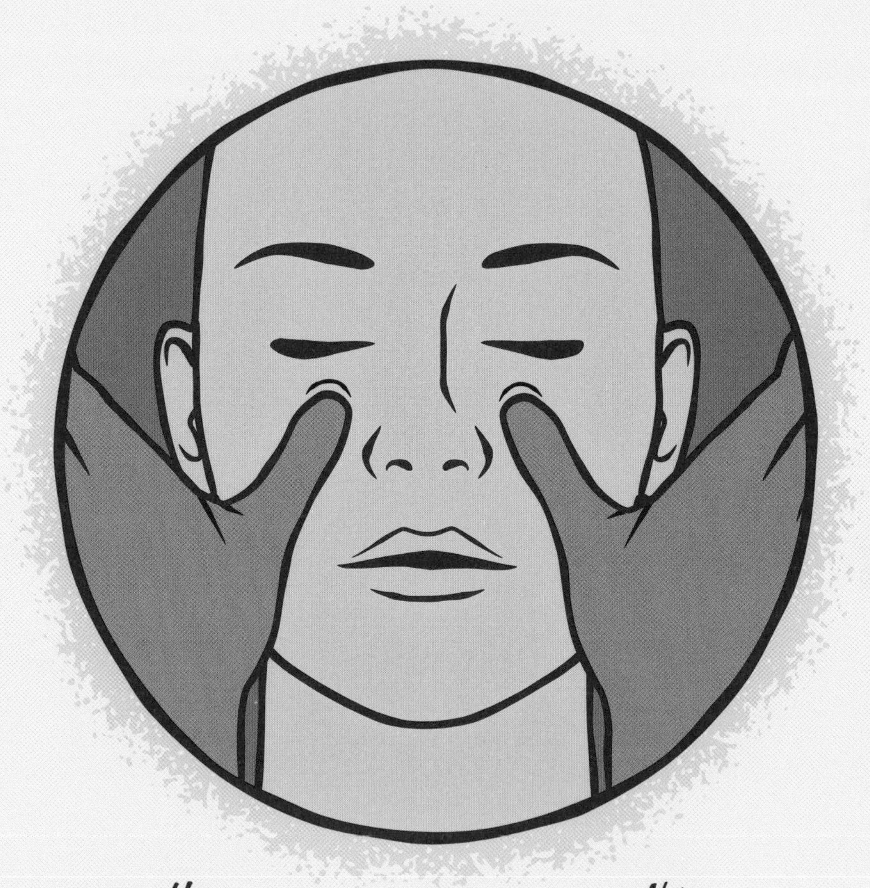

Uses

Helps with issues related to the eyes, as well as pain attributed to sinus infections and clogging.

Notes

This point can be used in place of ST 1, which should only be undertaken by practitioners with formal training.

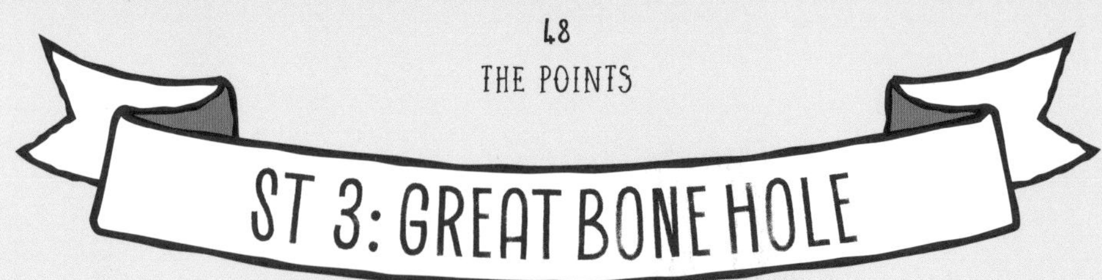

ST 3: GREAT BONE HOLE

Directly below the pupil in a depression 2 cun lateral of the nostrils.

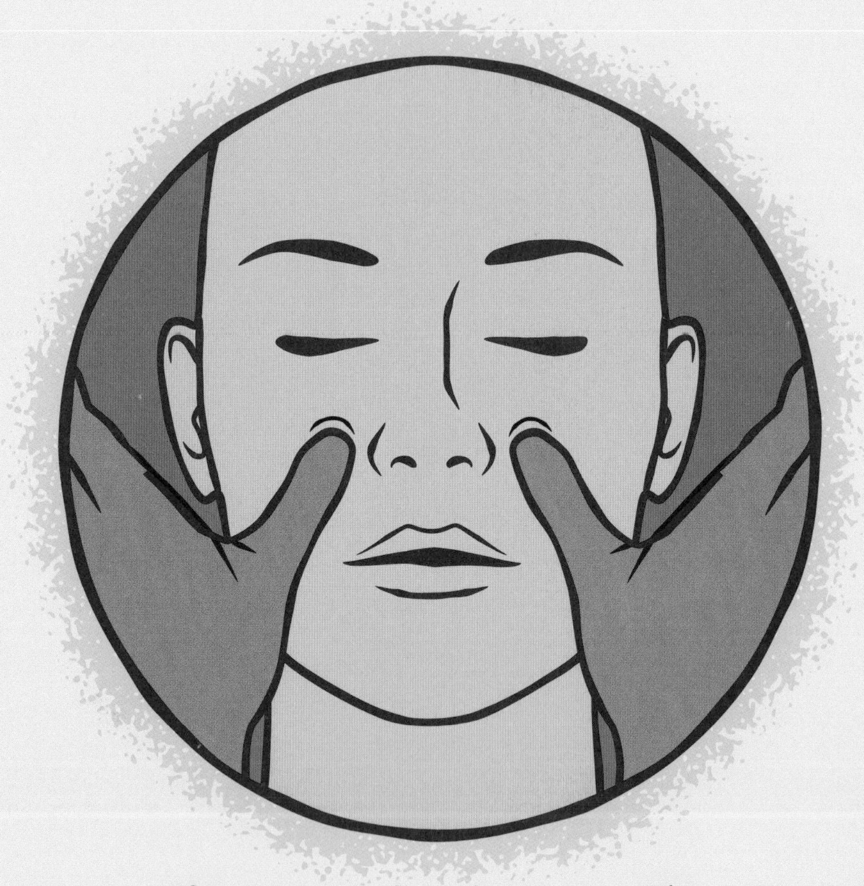

Uses

Used for facial paralysis, twitching of the eyes, and any issues related to pain attributed to sinus infections and clogging.

Notes

Use this point, along with ST 2 (see page 47), for sinus pain.

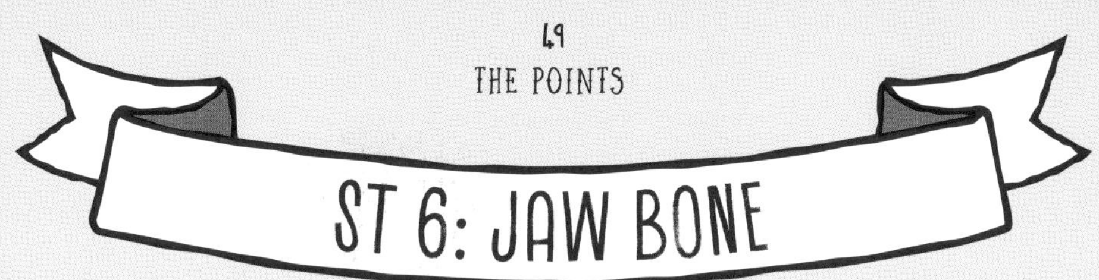

ST 6: JAW BONE

With clenched teeth, ST 6 is located in the belly of the masseter muscle, one finger's width anterior and superior to the angle of the mandible.

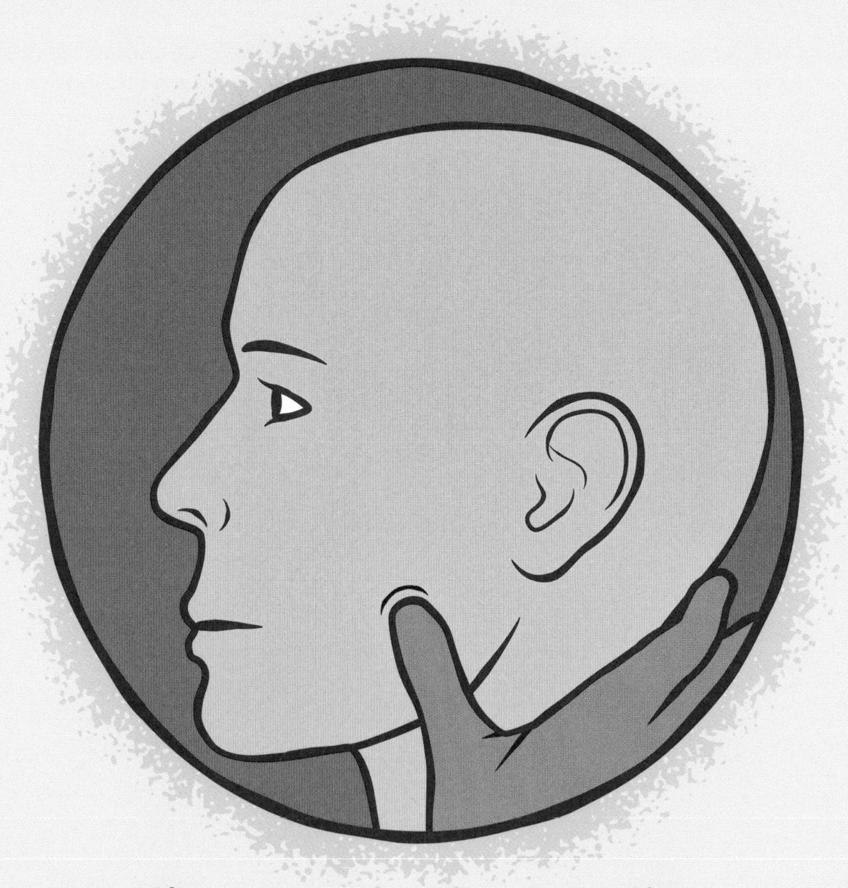

Uses

Commonly used for TMJD (temporomandibular joint disorder), toothache in the lower jaw, Bell's palsy, twitching, and facial pain or paralysis.

Notes

ST 6 is even said to help with a lost voice.

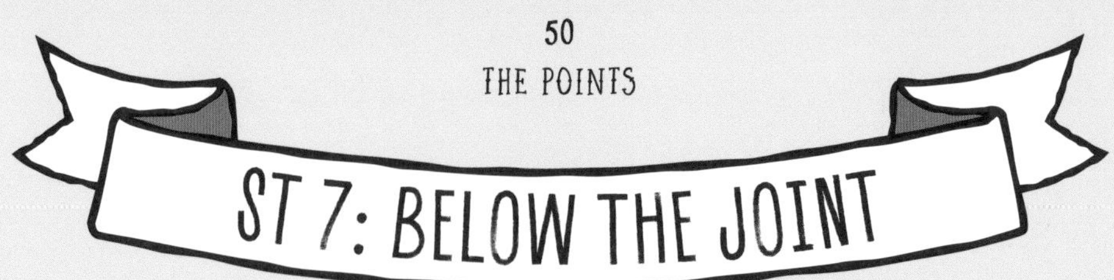

ST 7: BELOW THE JOINT

Located on the side of the face, anterior to the ear, in a depression between the zygomatic arch and the mandibular notch.

Uses

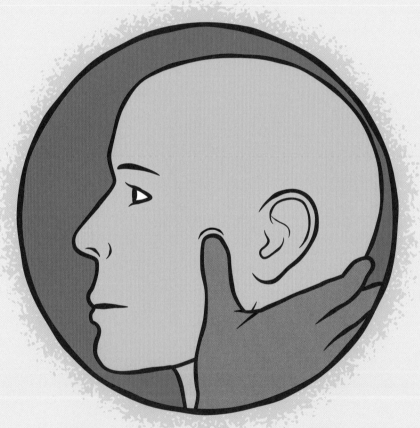

Used for any issues related to the ear, as well as TMJD (temporomandibular joint disorder), toothache, and nasal congestion.

Notes

When locating this point, be sure to keep the mouth closed.

ST 25: CELESTIAL PIVOT

On the abdomen, 2 cun lateral of the belly button on either side.

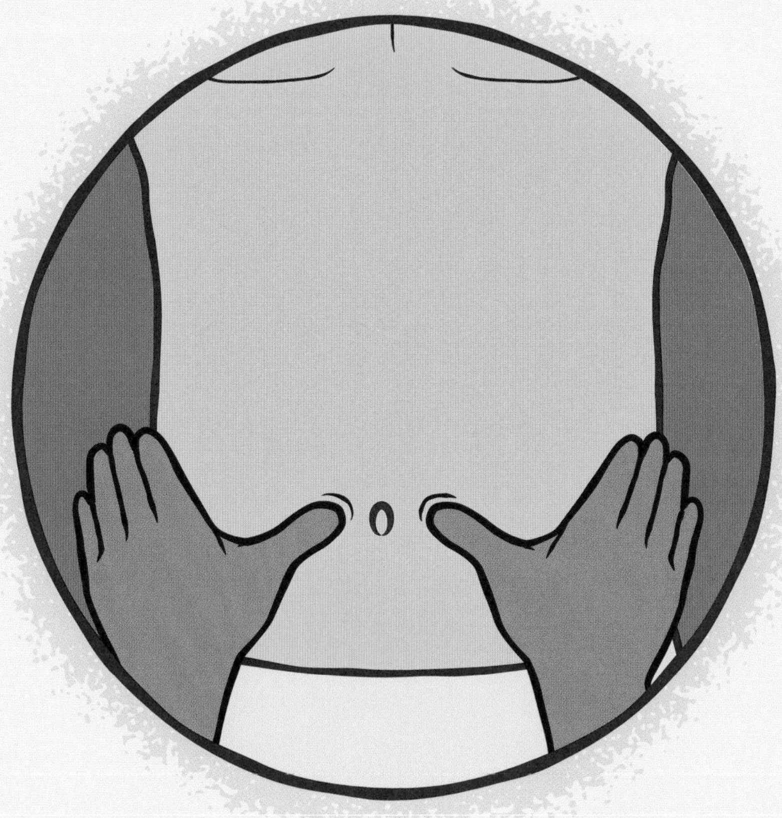

Uses

Helps with any issues in the lower digestive tract, as well as those related to menstruation and fertility.

Notes

This point may be used along with other ST points between the diaphragm and the top of the pelvis as part of a general abdominal/ female reproductive treatment.

ST 36: LEG THREE MILES

On the front side of the lower leg, 3 cun below the lower edge of the kneecap, in the depression 1 cun to the outside of the shin bone.

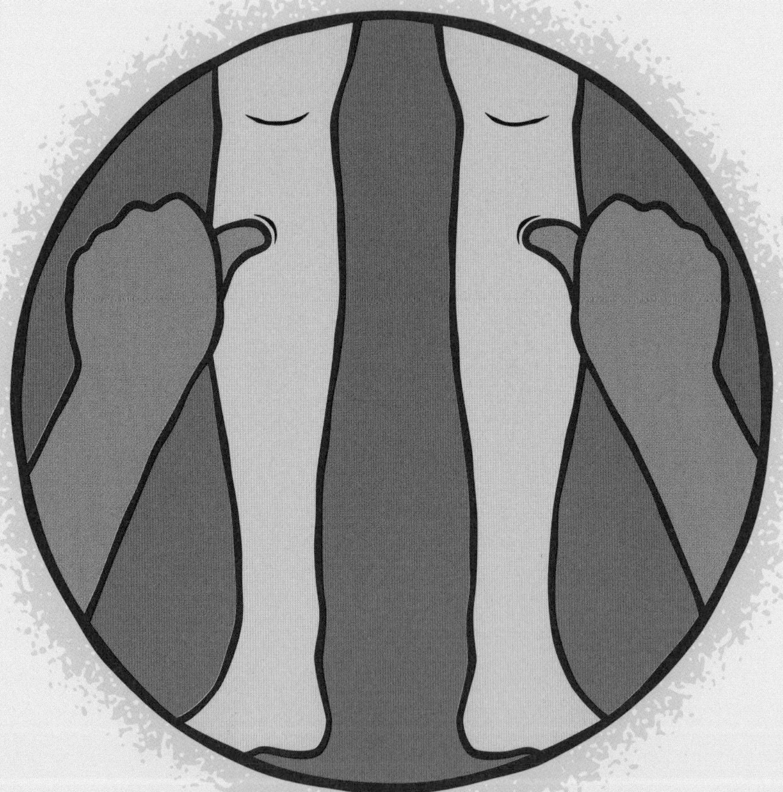

Uses

Relieves abdominal pain and digestive issues. Helps with leg pain, enhances qi and blood (see page 20), increases vitality while reducing fatigue, and helps calm the mind.

Notes

The word "miles" is a rough translation of the word *li* from the original Chinese name given for the point, *Zusanli*. Stimulating this point is said to invigorate the legs to such a degree that, even if fatigued, a person could walk another three miles.

ST 37: UPPER GREAT HOLLOW

On the front side of the lower leg, 6 cun below the lower edge of the kneecap, in the depression 1 cun to the outside of the shin bone.

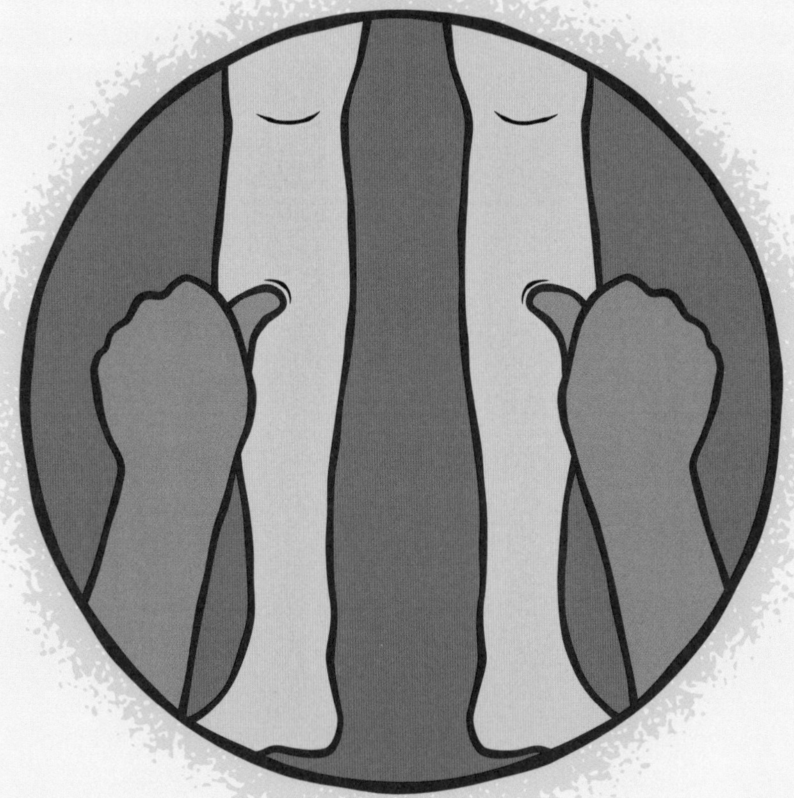

Uses

Used for acute disorders of the intestines and digestive system, including diarrhea, constipation, bloating, gurgling, and general abdominal pain.

Notes

ST 37 is a good point for resolving issues of Damp-Heat (see page 20).

SP 6: THREE YIN INTERSECTION

On the inside of the lower leg, 3 cun above the upper edge of the ankle, in the depression off the back of the shin bone.

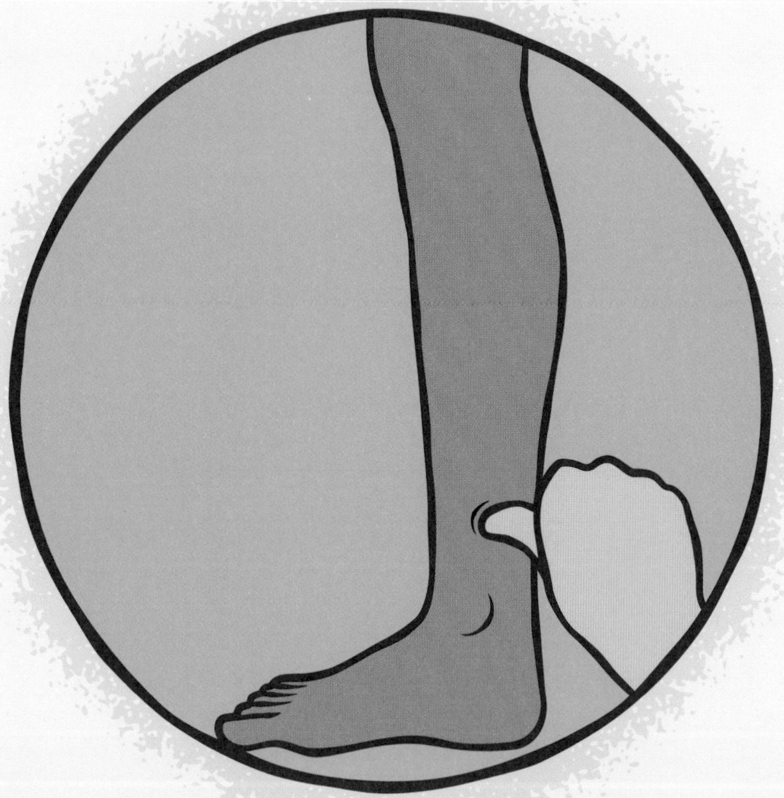

Uses

Can provide general relaxation and help with insomnia and issues related to anxiety. Helps to stimulate digestion and is especially useful for issues related to the female reproductive system.

Notes

One of the most common points you will come across, SP 6 is known for dealing with emotional, digestive, and gynecological issues. The name derives from the placement of SP 6 at the intersection of three meridians (Spleen, Kidney, and Liver). **Not to be used during pregnancy.**

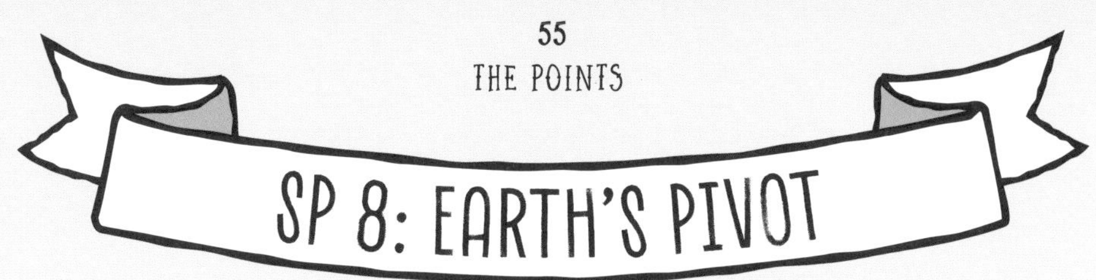

SP 8: EARTH'S PIVOT

Located on the inside of the lower leg, 3 cun below SP 9 (see page 56).

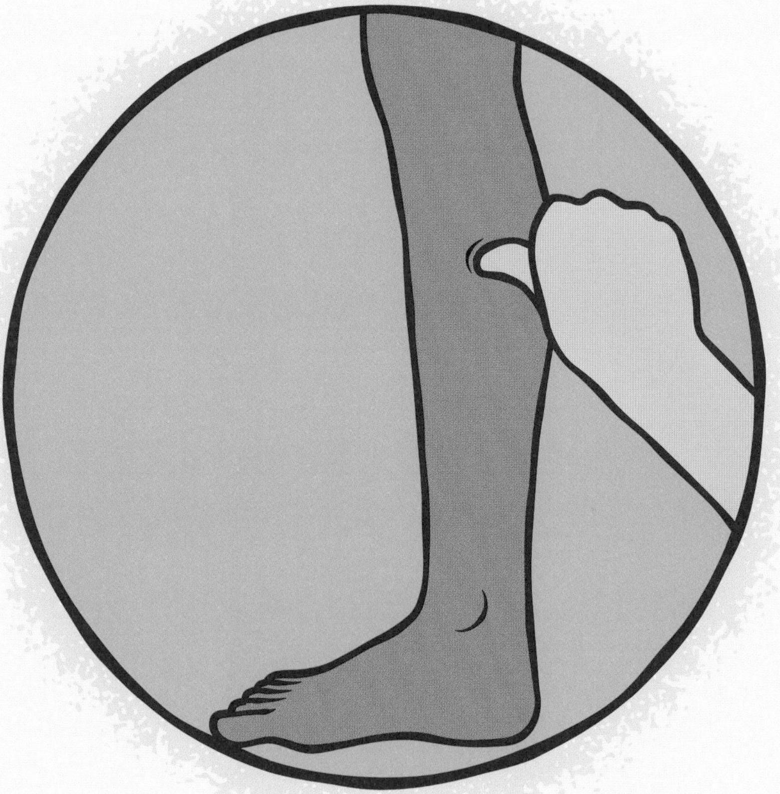

Uses

Often used for acute and painful menstrual issues due to blood stagnation, including clotting, fibroids, dysmenorrhea, and irregular menstruation. Also used for treating diarrhea.

Notes

SP 8 may also be used for issues relating to male infertility, such as seminal emission and depleted sex drive.

SP 9: YIN MOUND SPRING

Located on the inside of the lower leg, in the depression at the lower border of the medial condyle of the tibia.

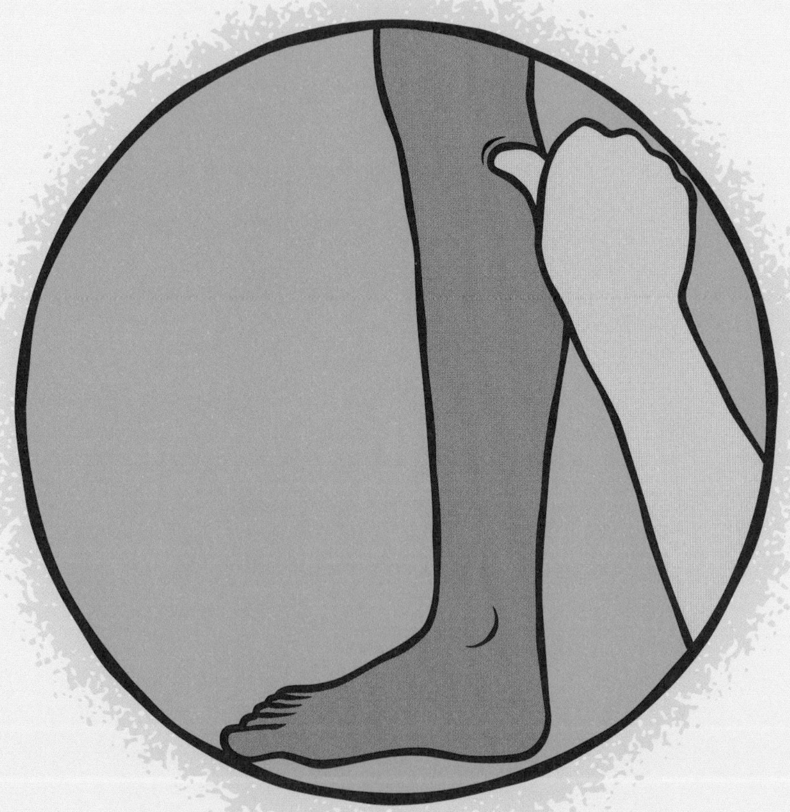

Uses

Used for abdominal issues, including diarrhea, bloating, and swelling, and also urinary issues.

Notes

SP 9 is considered to be one of the most important, if not the most important, points for dealing with Dampness (see page 21) in the abdominal region of the body.

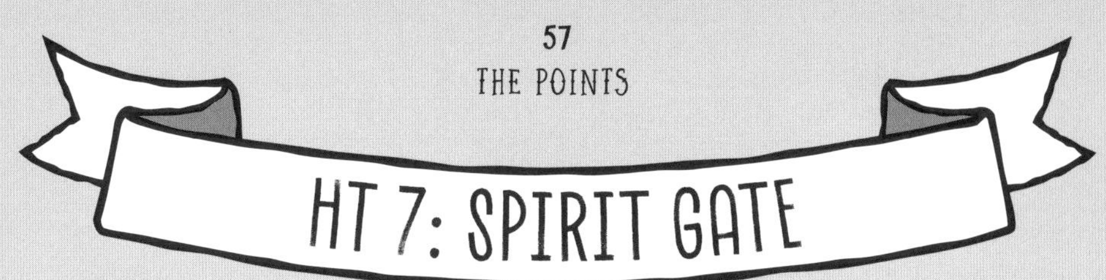

HT 7: SPIRIT GATE

Located in a depression on the pinky side of the wrist crease.

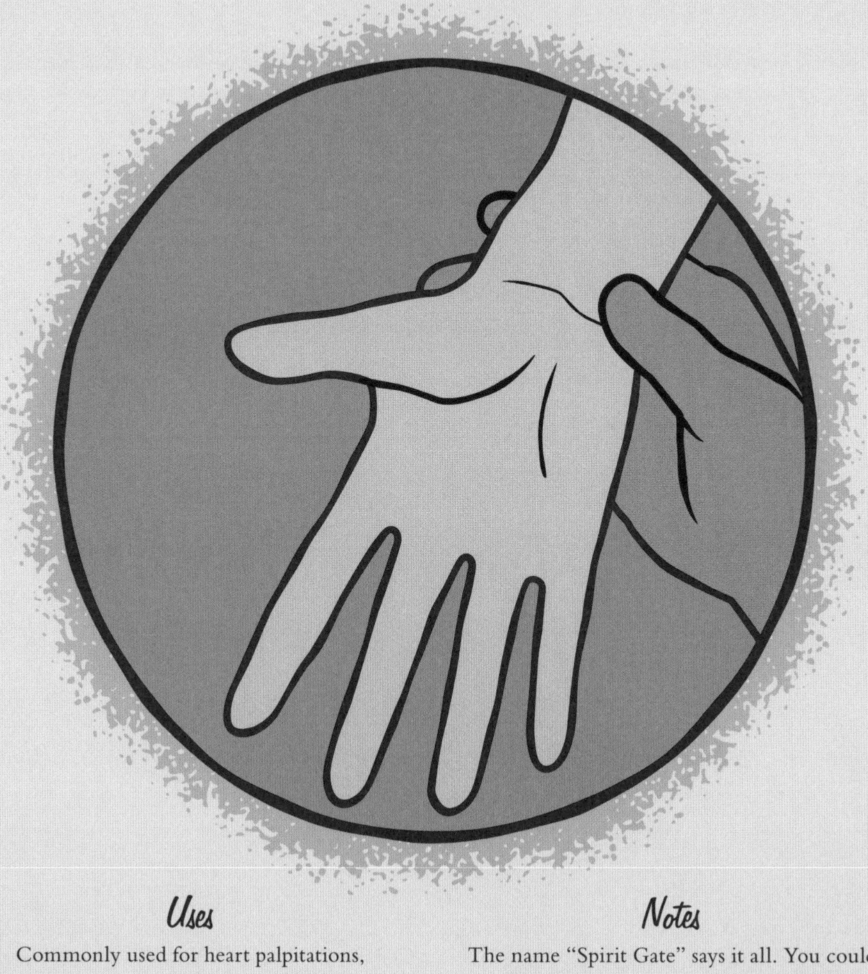

Uses

Commonly used for heart palpitations, anxiety, emotional issues, and insomnia.

Notes

The name "Spirit Gate" says it all. You could think of HT 7 as a significant point for calming the spirit or mind.

SI 11: CELESTIAL GATHERING

Located in a depression in the middle of the scapulae, or shoulder blades.

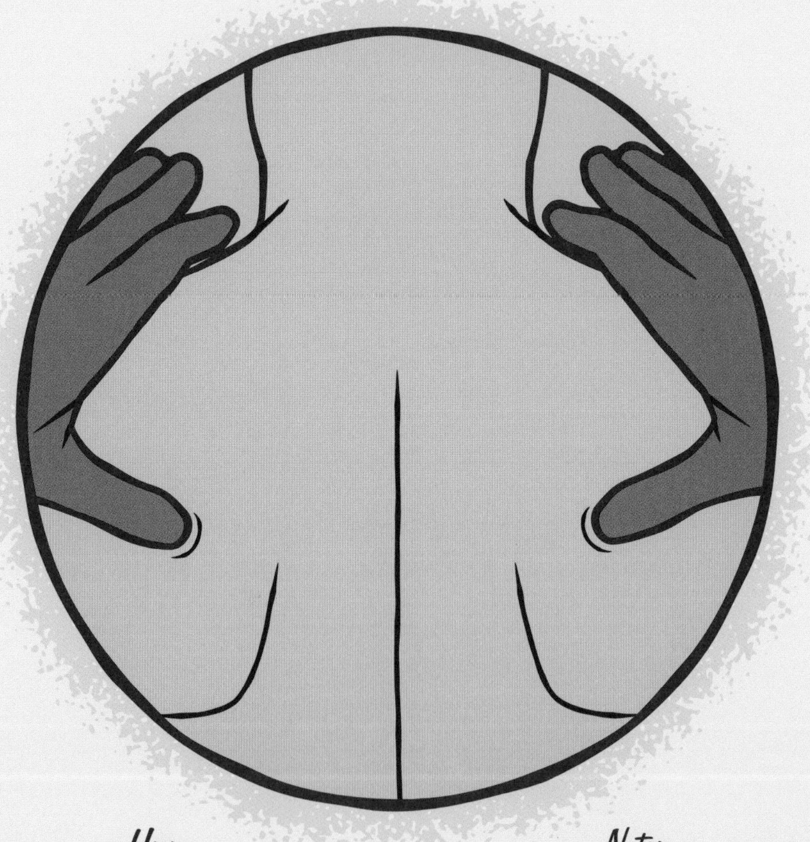

Uses

Commonly used as a local point for shoulder pain and pain patterns in the arms, as well as emotional issues such as anxiety and depression.

Notes

SI 11 is also commonly used for breast-related issues, such as mastitis, insufficient lactation, and breast pain.

SI 19: HEARING PALACE

Located in the depression formed when the mouth is open, anterior to the tragus and posterior to the condyloid process of the mandible.

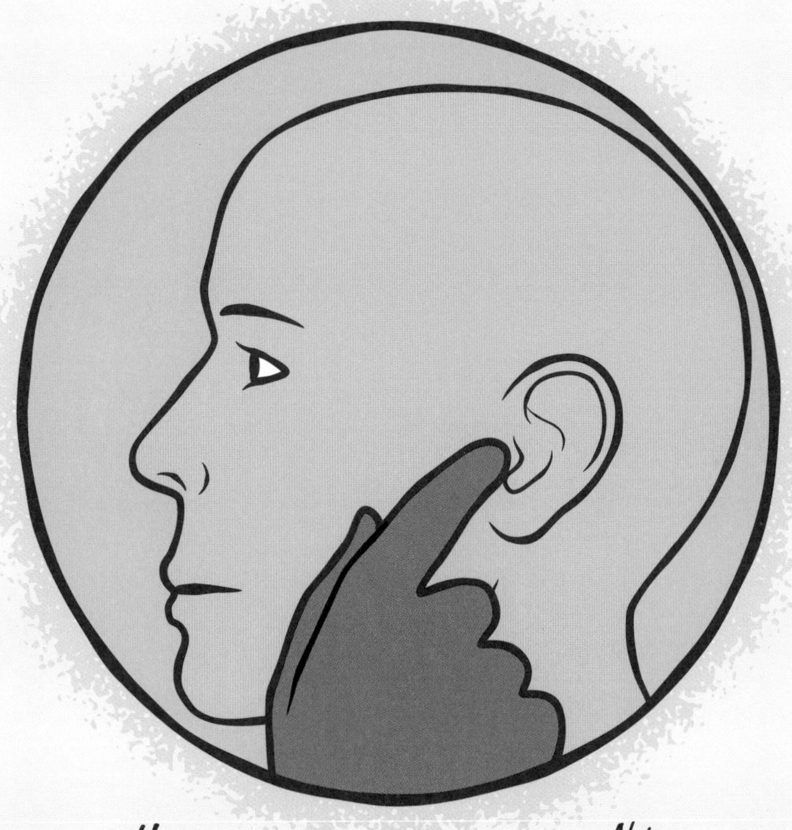

Uses

SI 19 is primarily used for ear problems such as inflammation, deafness, tinnitus, and hearing loss. It is also used for TMJD (temporomandibular joint disorder) and general issues related to toothache.

Notes

Like HT 7 (see page 57), SI 19 is known to calm the spirit.

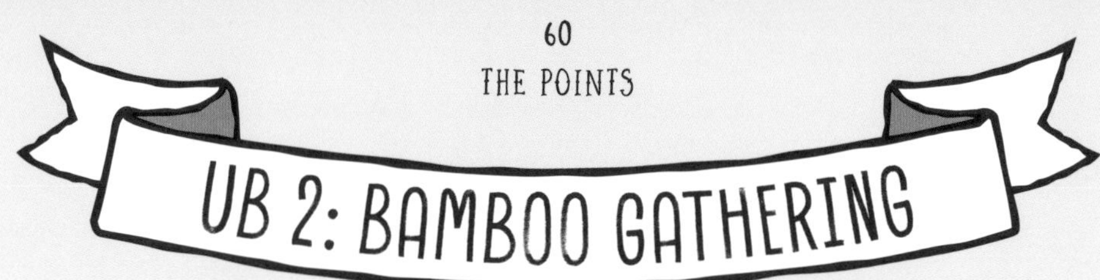

UB 2: BAMBOO GATHERING

Located in the depression at the medial border of the eyebrows.

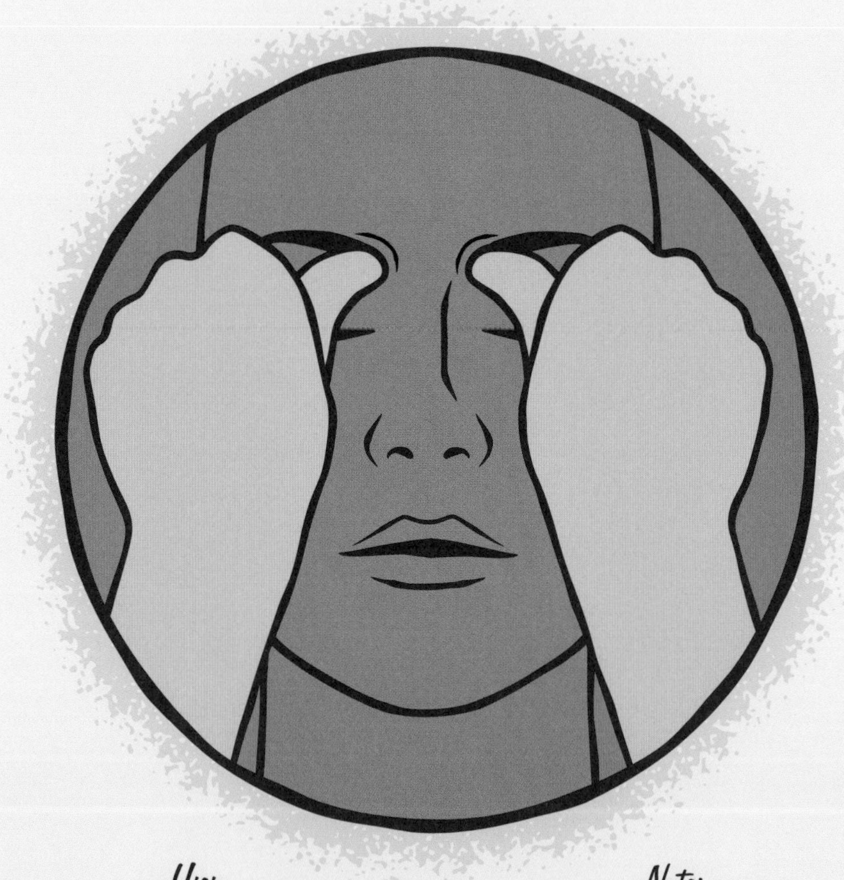

Uses

Used to treat sinus congestion, headaches, and allergy symptoms associated with the eyes.

Notes

This is a commonly used point when massaging the face.

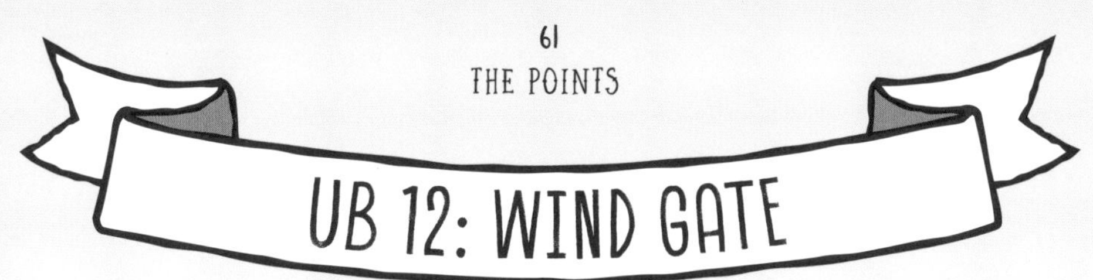

UB 12: WIND GATE

Located 1.5 cun lateral to the second thoracic vertebra.

Uses

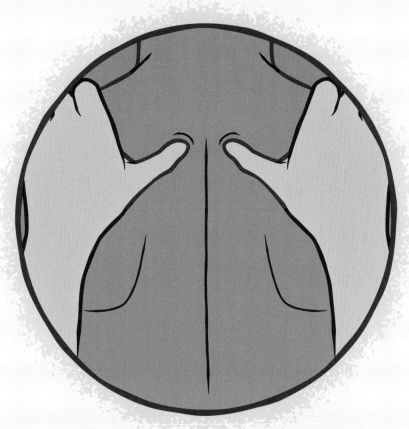

Used to treat early stages of a cold, and help relieve coughing and fever.

Notes

UB 12 used with ST 36 (see page 52) can help build up a defense against colds that penetrate deep into the body.

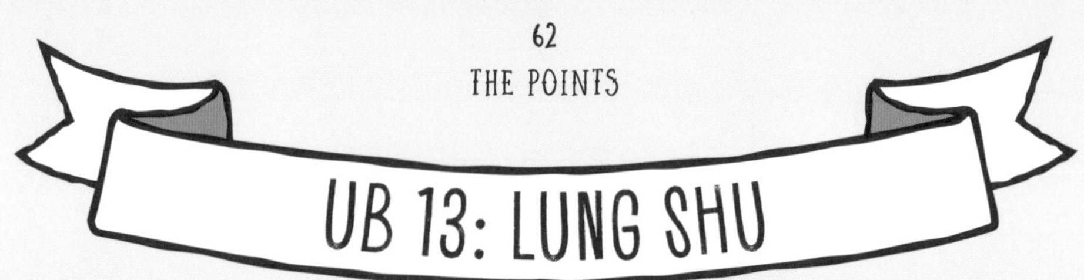

UB 13: LUNG SHU

Located 1.5 cun lateral to the third thoracic vertebra.

Uses

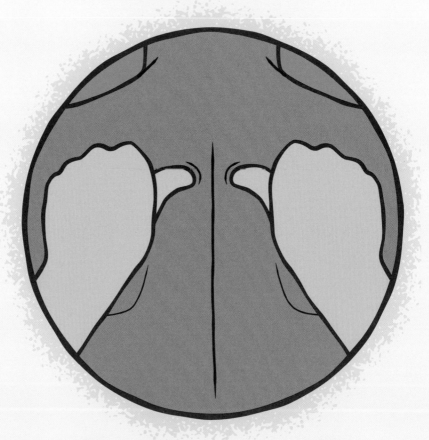

Used to treat many issues related to colds affecting the lungs, including coughing, congestion, asthma, wheezing, shortness of breath, and weakness in vocal projection.

Notes

In Traditional Chinese Medicine, the lung is associated with grief and sadness. As UB 13 is the main point for all lung issues, it may be used to help with these emotional states.

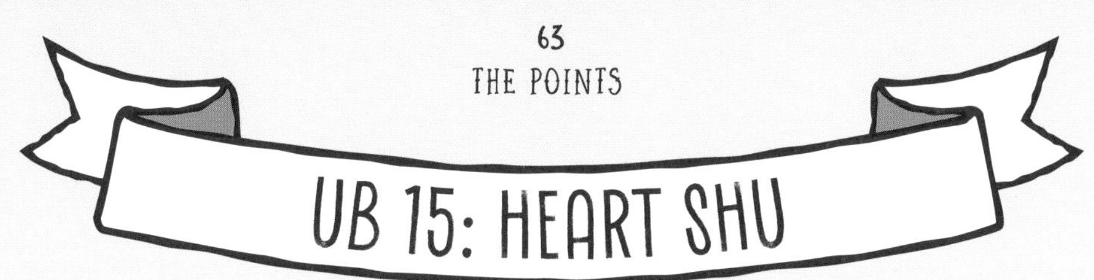

UB 15: HEART SHU

Located 1.5 cun lateral to the fifth thoracic vertebra.

Uses

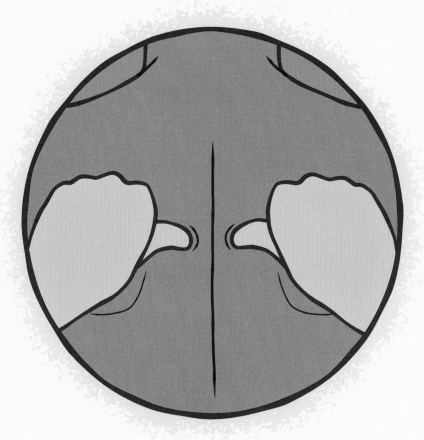

Since it is related to the heart, UB 15 may be used for cardiac pain, heart palpitations, chest congestion, shortness of breath, and coughing. It is also used for insomnia, forgetfulness, and epilepsy.

Notes

UB 15 is known as one of the most important points to consider when working with insomnia and anxiety.

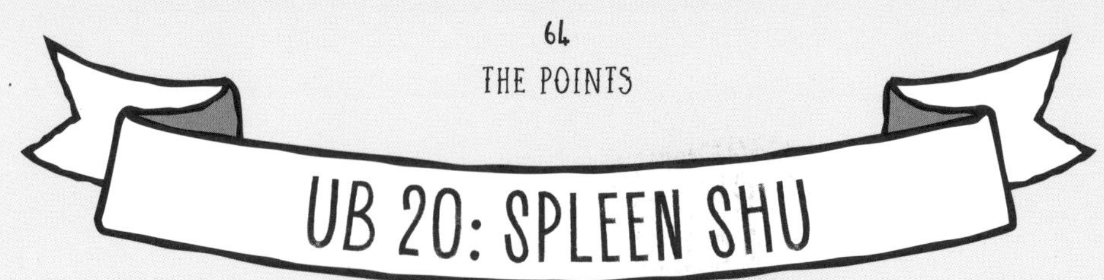

UB 20: SPLEEN SHU

Located 1.5 cun lateral to the eleventh thoracic vertebra.

Uses

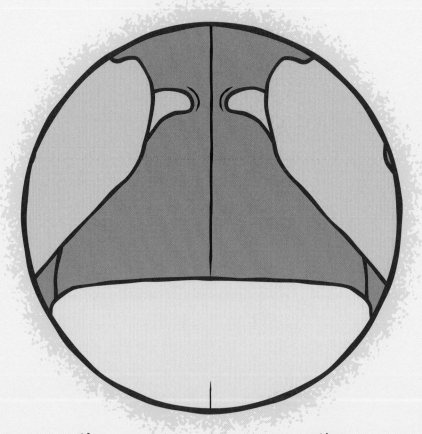

Used to treat issues within the abdominal region, including diarrhea, distention, bloating, and abdominal pain.

Notes

UB 20 is a commonly used point for all issues related to the TCM (Traditional Chinese Medicine) understanding of the spleen.

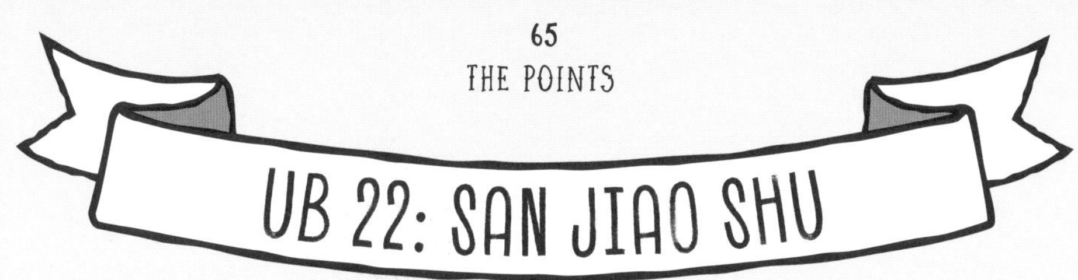

UB 22: SAN JIAO SHU

Located 1.5 cun lateral to the first lumbar vertebra.

Uses

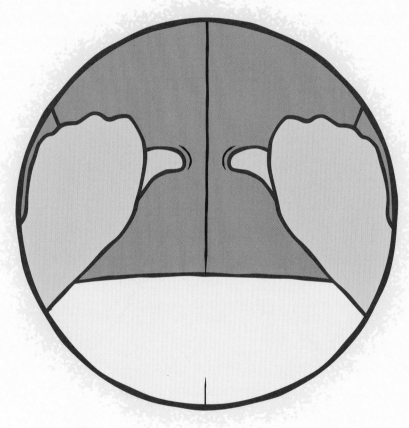

Commonly used for distention of the abdomen, gurgling in the belly, and diarrhea.

Notes

UB 22 is commonly used for issues related to Dampness (see page 21).

UB 25: LARGE INTESTINE SHU

Located 1.5 cun lateral to the fourth lumbar vertebra.

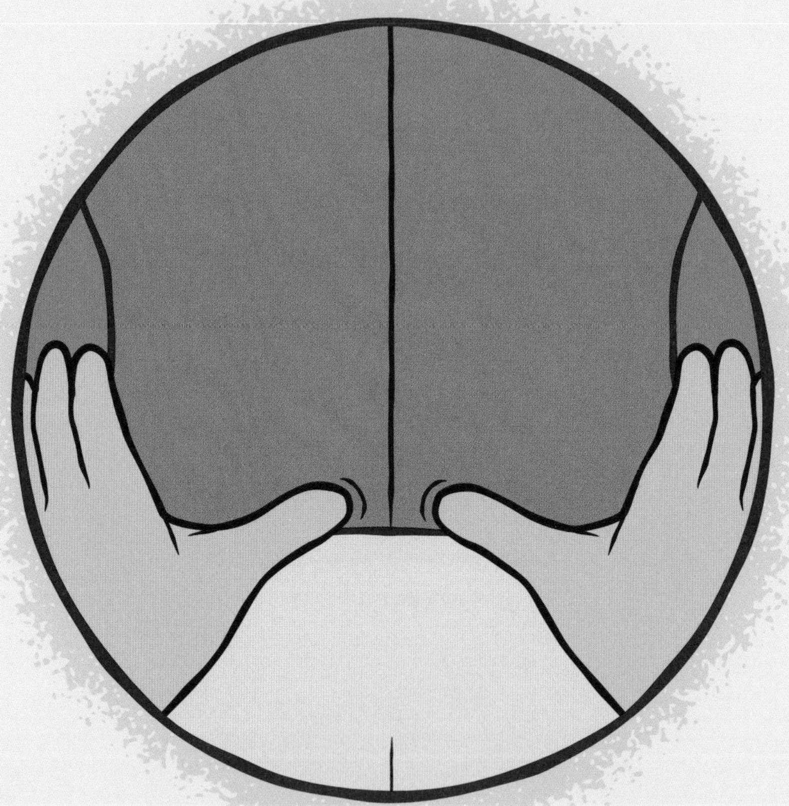

Uses

Commonly used for abdominal distention, diarrhea, and constipation, as well as lumbar pain.

Notes

UB 25 is a very common point for constipation and diarrhea. Its physical location also makes this point particularly useful when dealing with lower back pain.

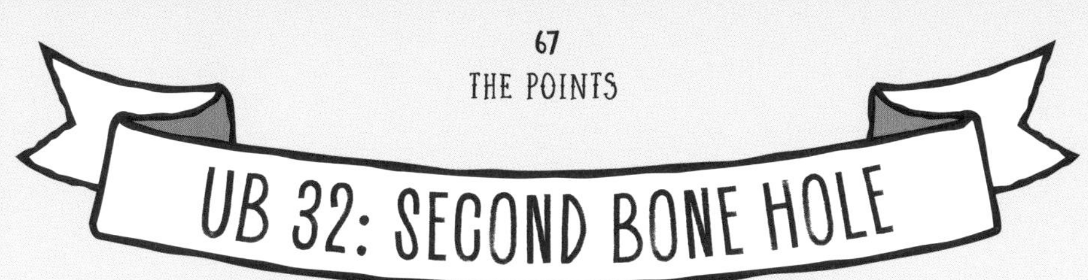

UB 32: SECOND BONE HOLE

Located in the second sacral foramen.

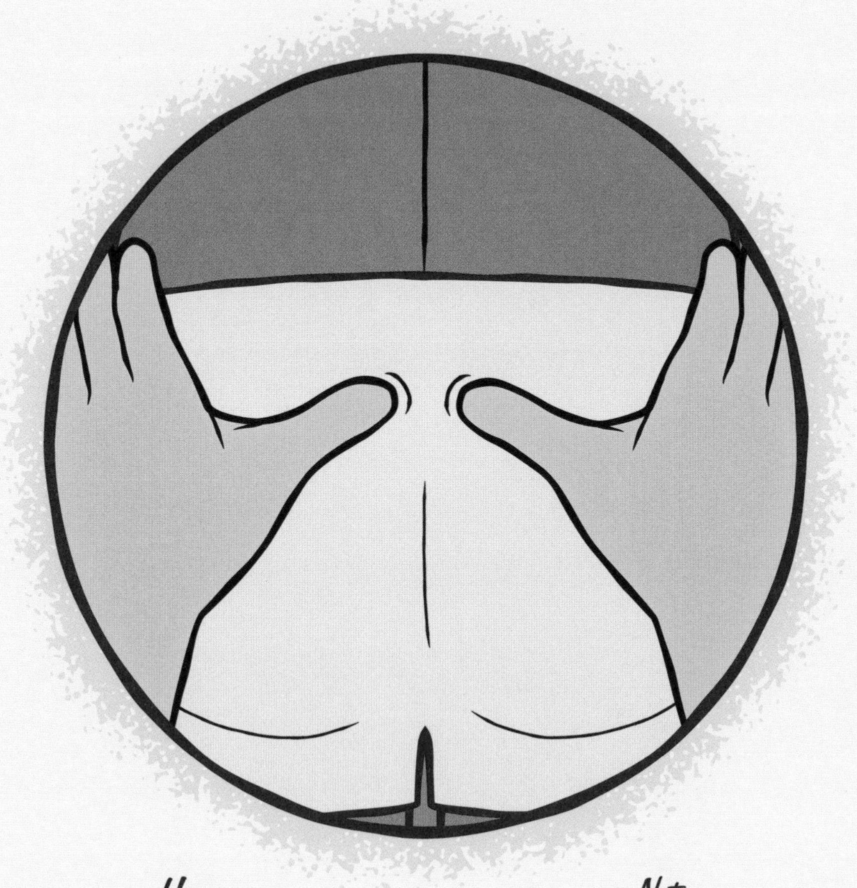

Uses

Commonly used for lumbosacral and lower abdominal pain, as well as for issues related to the uterus.

Notes

UB 32 is the most commonly used of the four sacral foramen points, together known as the Eight Liao, which are often indicated for local lower back or sacral issues, as well as for many genital and urinary-related conditions. Also helps with regaining mobility in the lower limbs.

UB 40: BEND MIDDLE

Located in the middle of the crease behind the knee between the lower hamstring attachments.

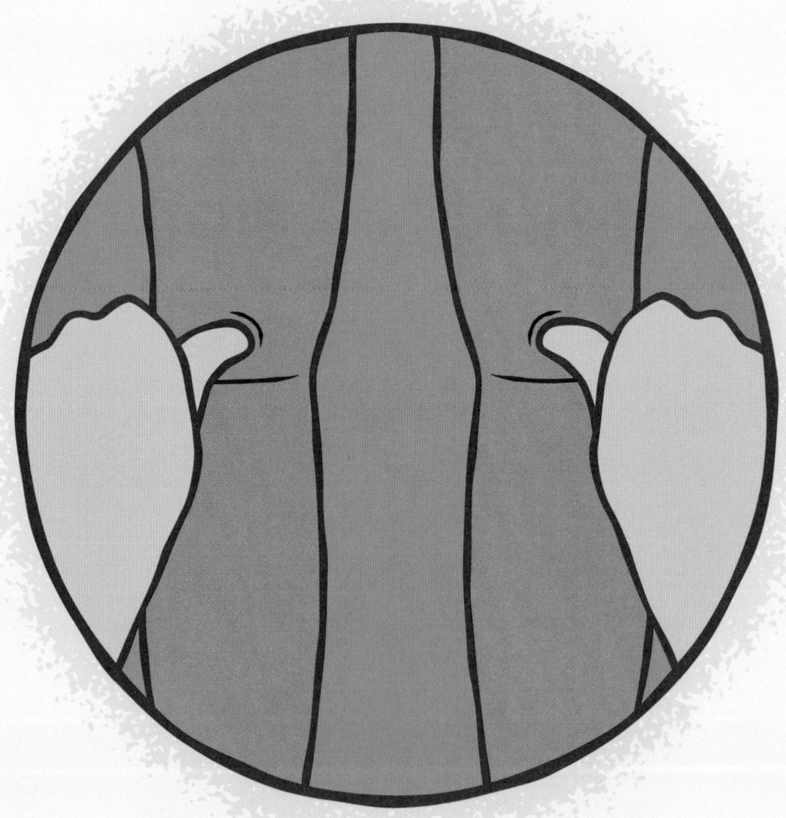

Uses

Known as the Lumbar Command Point, UB 40 is commonly used for lumbar-related issues.

Notes

UB 40 is one of the most popular points for lower back pain.

UB 60: KUNLUN MOUNTAINS

Outside of the lower leg at the level of the tip of the ankle bone, in the depression between the ankle and the Achilles tendon.

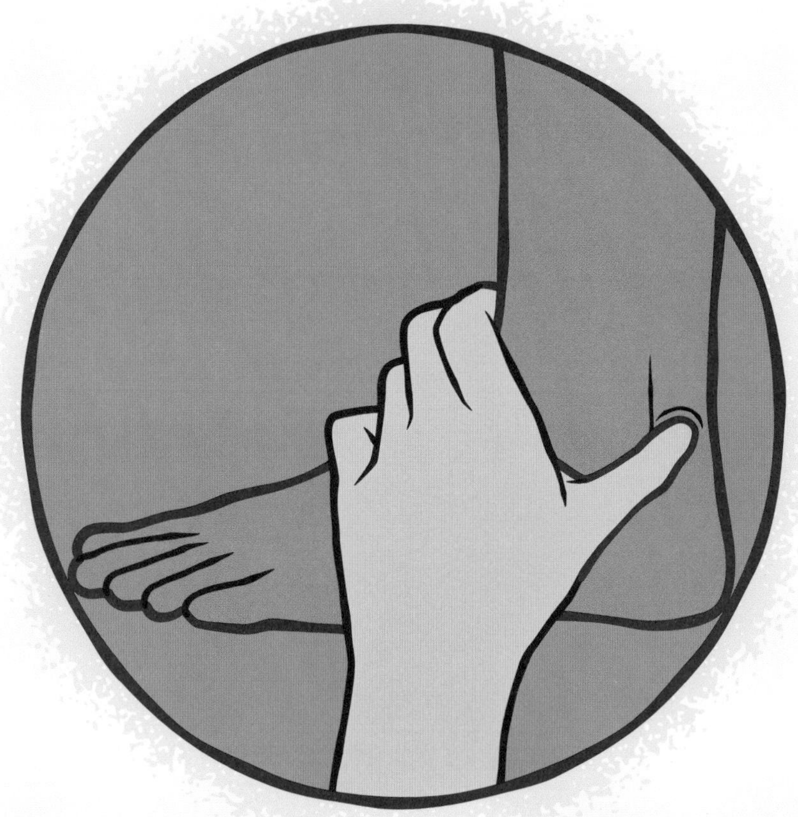

Uses

Relieves pain along the spine, and especially in the lower back. Helps with headaches and neck pain.

Notes

UB 60 is considered a significant point to help with difficult labor, but is contraindicated during the natural pregnancy cycle. **Not to be used during pregnancy.**

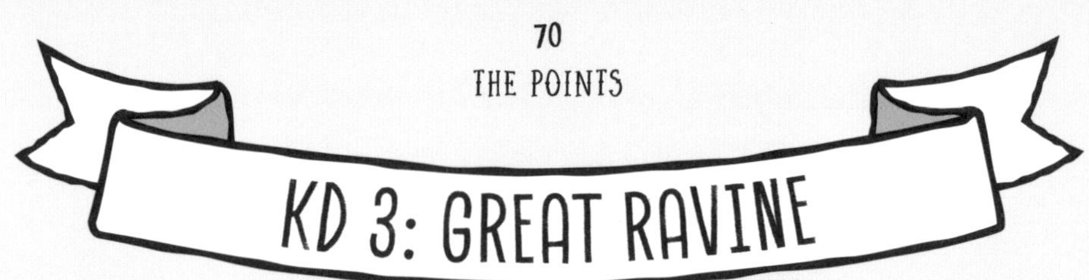

KD 3: GREAT RAVINE

Located in the depression at the level of the ankle on the inside of the leg.

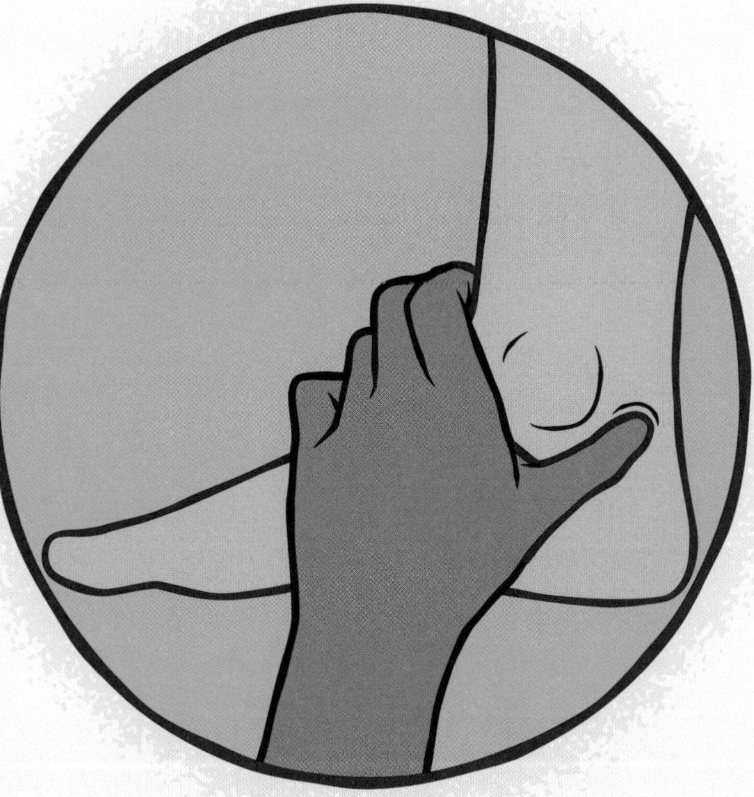

Uses

Used for difficulty inhaling in association with asthma, as well as impotence, frequent urination, irregular menstruation, and lower back pain.

Notes

KD 3 is an important point for all deficient kidney patterns (see page 21).

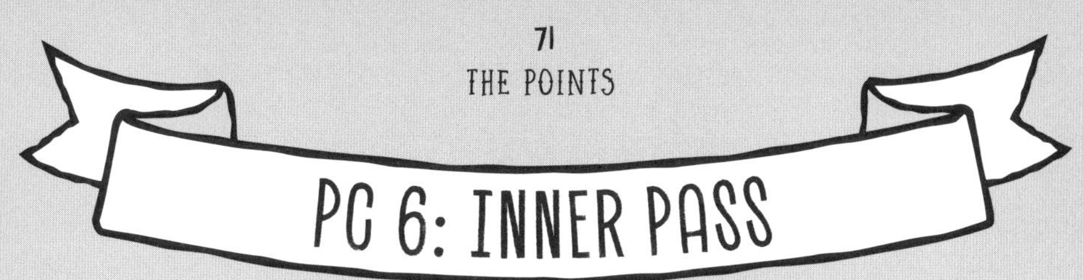

PC 6: INNER PASS

Located on the inside of the arm 2 cun above the middle of the wrist.

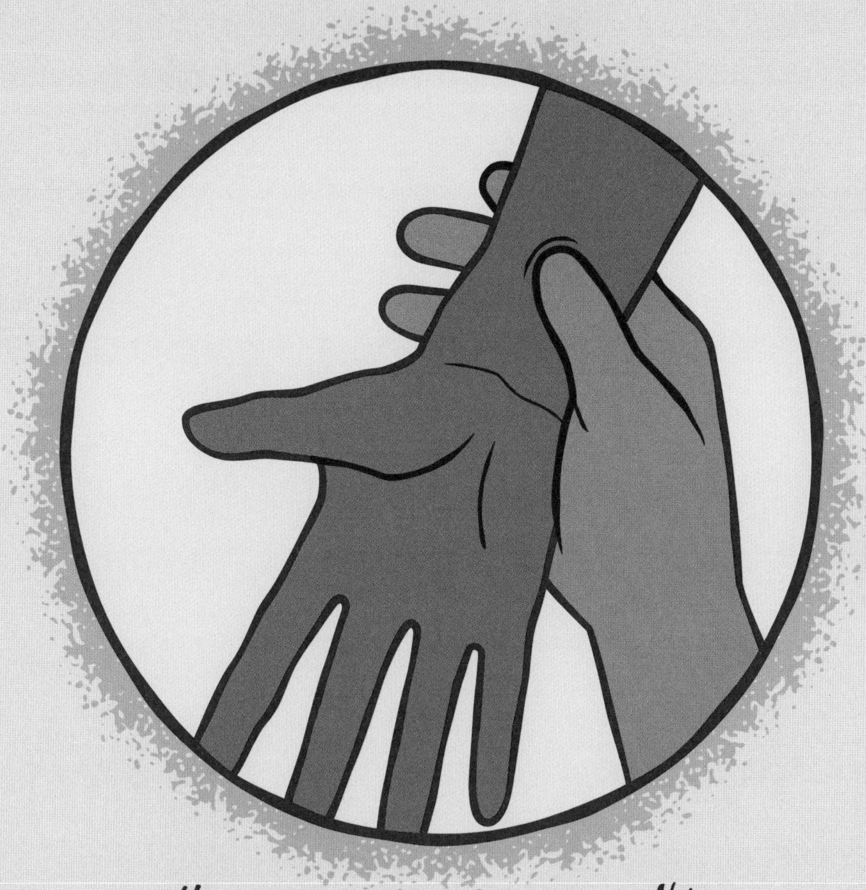

Uses

Congestion in the chest, nausea, sea and motion sickness, vomiting, and insomnia.

Notes

One of the most commonly used points, PC 6 is also known to calm the mind.

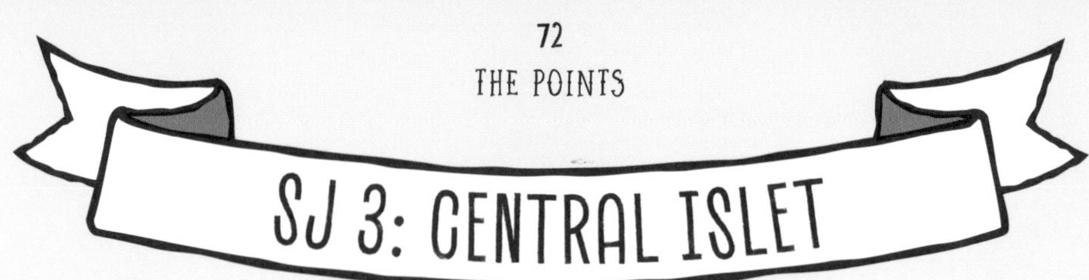

SJ 3: CENTRAL ISLET

Located in a depression on the dorsum of the hand between the fourth and fifth metacarpal bones.

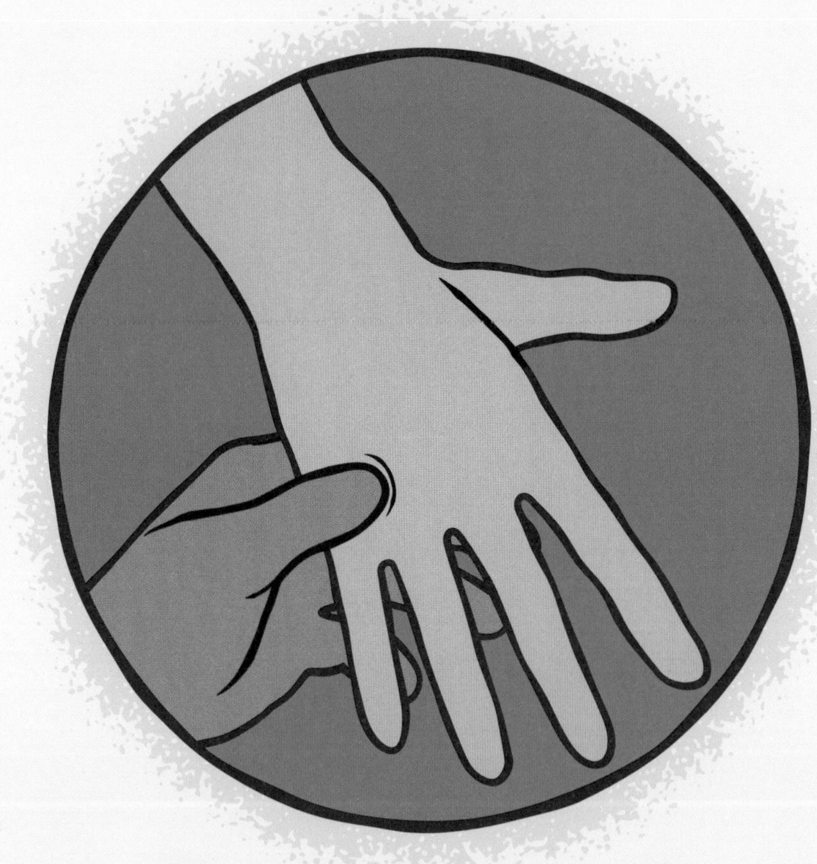

Uses

Most issues related to the ear, as well as headaches, pain around the shoulder and scapula, and sore throat.

Notes

SJ 3 may be used for pain or tension held in the joints.

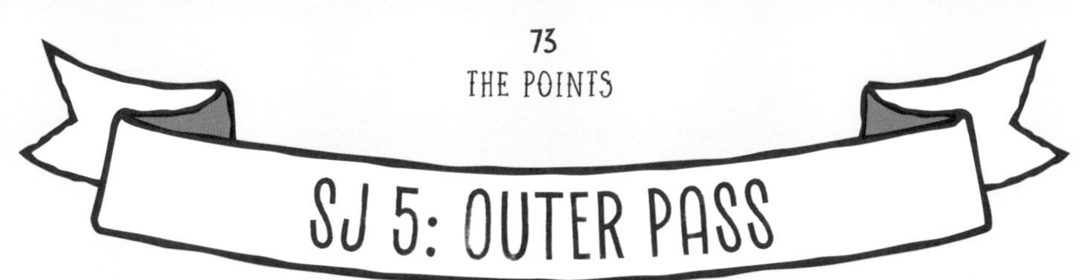

SJ 5: OUTER PASS

Located in a depression on the back of the arm between the ulna and radius, 2 cun above the crease in the wrist.

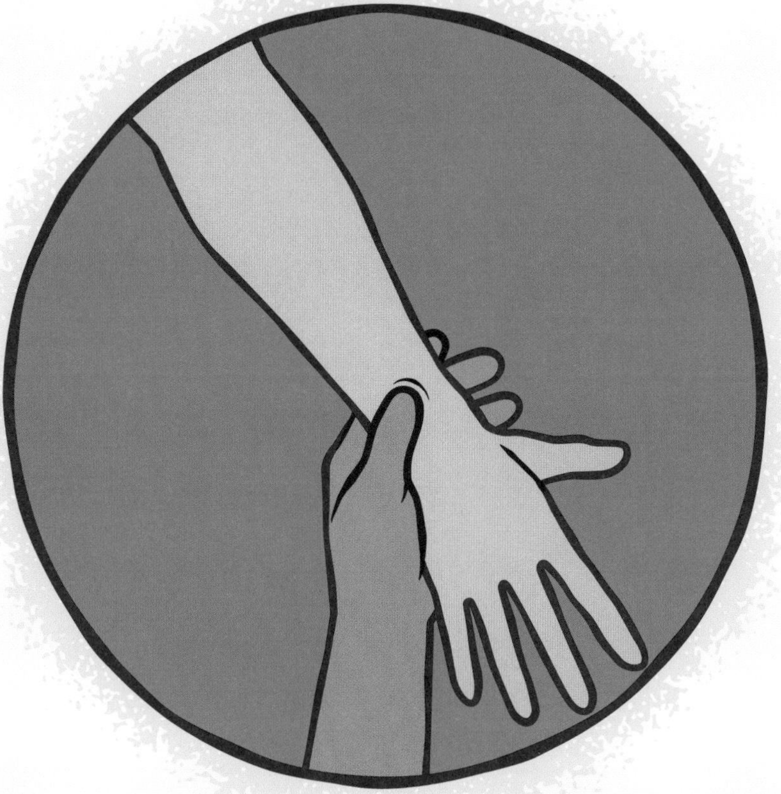

Uses

Used for pain associated with headaches and migraines, as well as general arm pains.

Notes

Very useful point for releasing exterior Wind-Heat (see page 20).

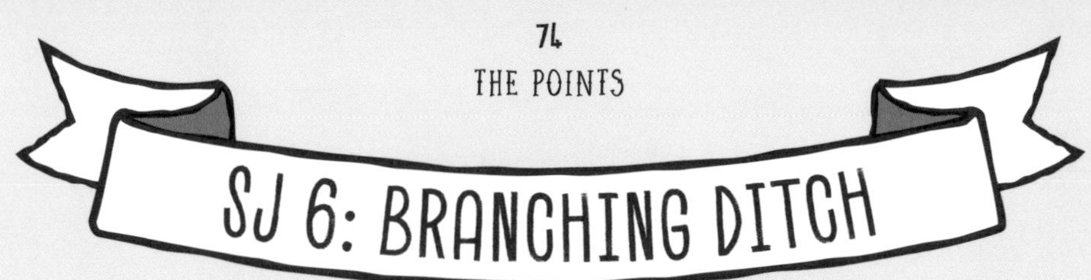

SJ 6: BRANCHING DITCH

Located in a depression on the back of the arm between the ulna and radius, 3 cun above the crease in the wrist.

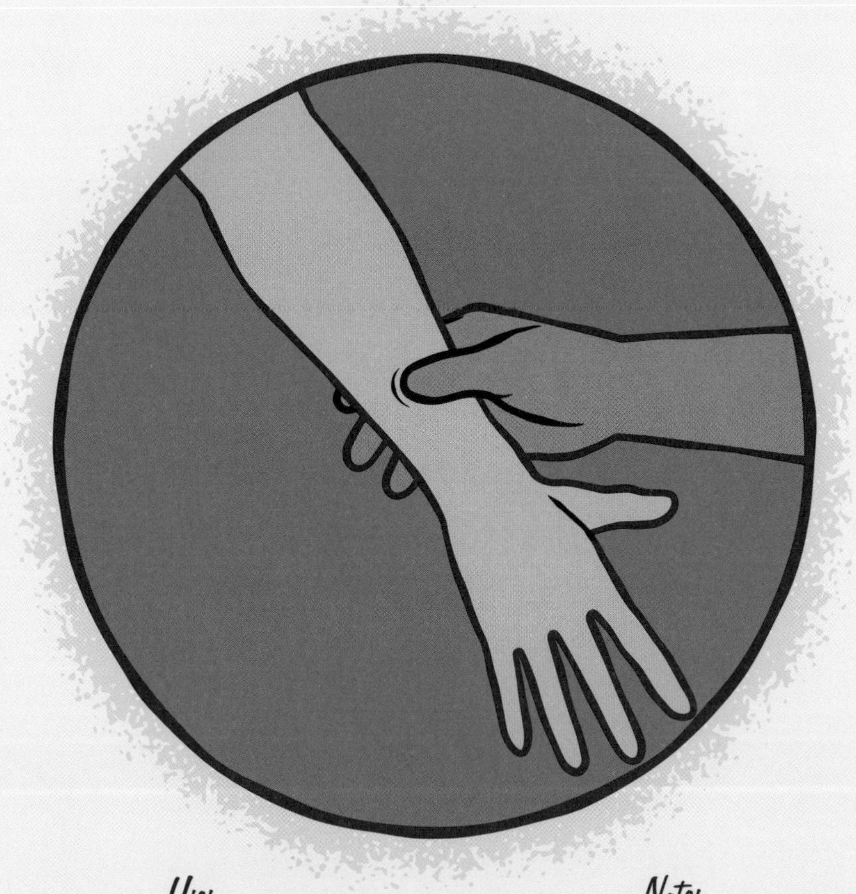

Uses

Used for constipation due to stagnation and Heat (see page 20).

Notes

Can also be used as part of a treatment for sudden bouts of vomiting or diarrhea.

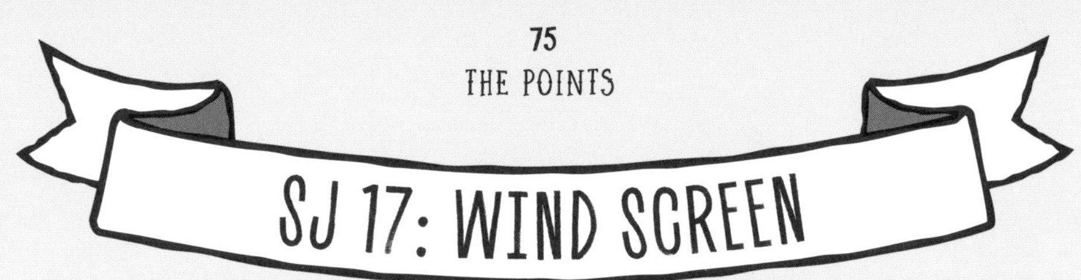

SJ 17: WIND SCREEN

Located in a depression behind the earlobe between the angle of the mandible and the mastoid process.

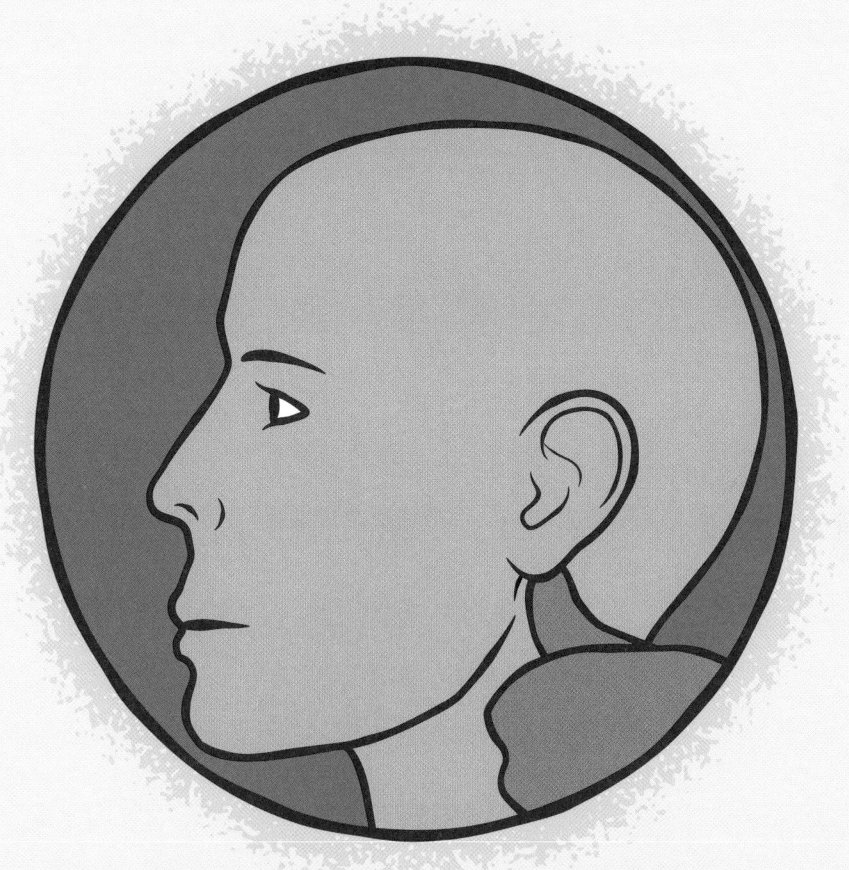

Uses

Used for earaches, tinnitus, and toothache.

Notes

SJ 17 is known to disperse Wind while clearing Heat (see page 20). SJ 17 benefits the head and face, and alleviates pain.

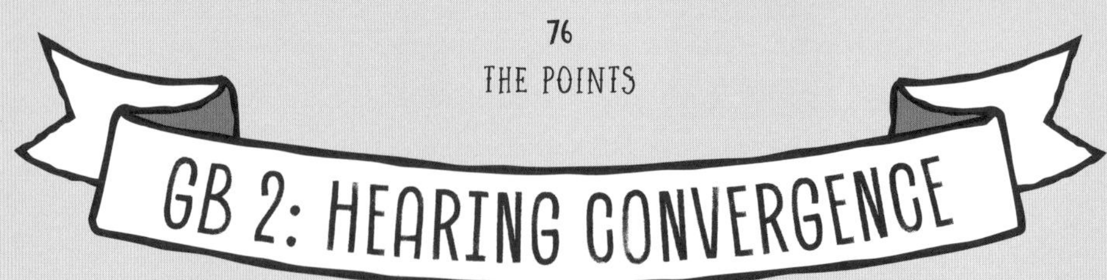

GB 2: HEARING CONVERGENCE

When the mouth is open, located in a depression in front of the tragus notch and behind the condyloid process of the mandible.

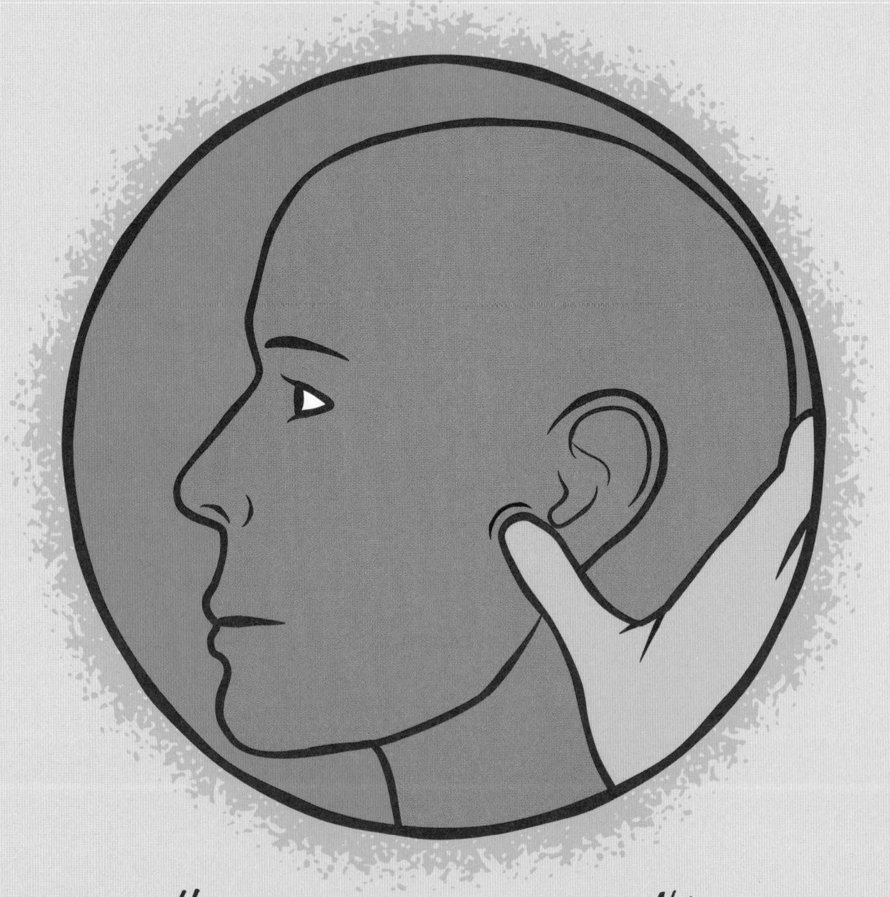

Uses

Used for issues related to the ear, as well as toothache and TMJD (temporomandibular joint disorder).

Notes

Be sure to differentiate between GB 2 and SI 19 (see page 59), which are very close together.

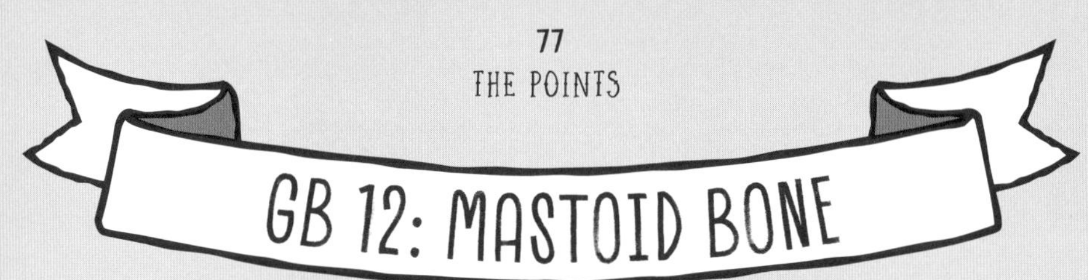

GB 12: MASTOID BONE

Found behind the ear in a depression posterior and inferior to the mastoid process.

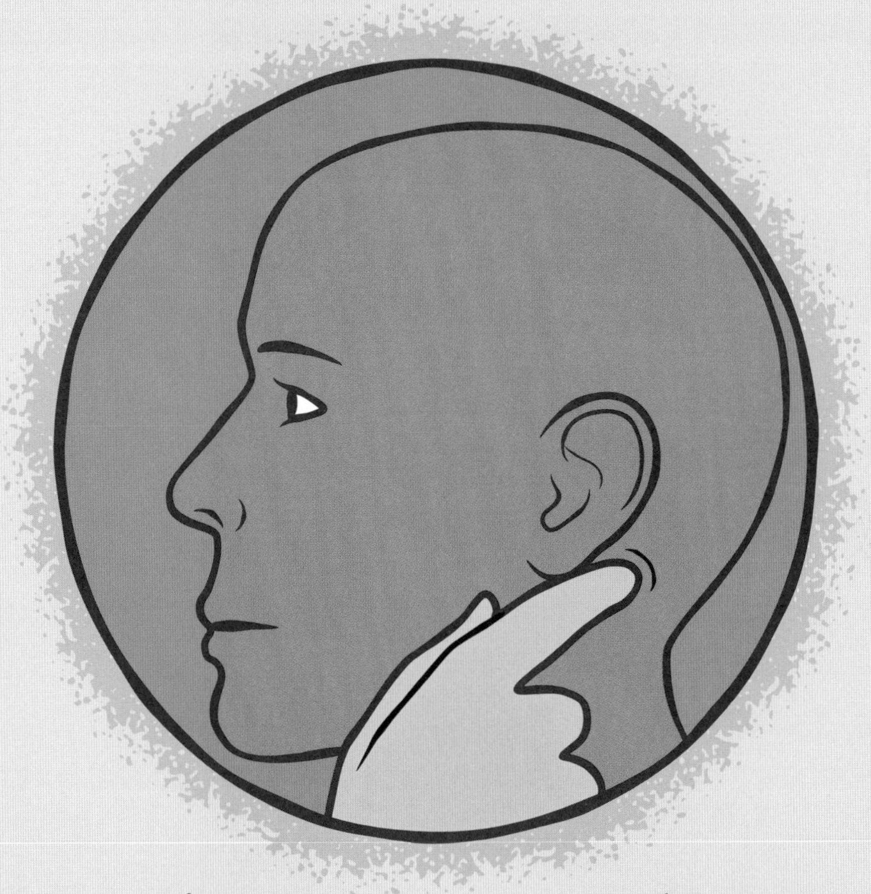

Uses

GB 12 is a great point for jaw pain, headaches, stiff necks, and toothache.

Notes

GB 12 is also said to calm the spirit and help with anxiety and insomnia.

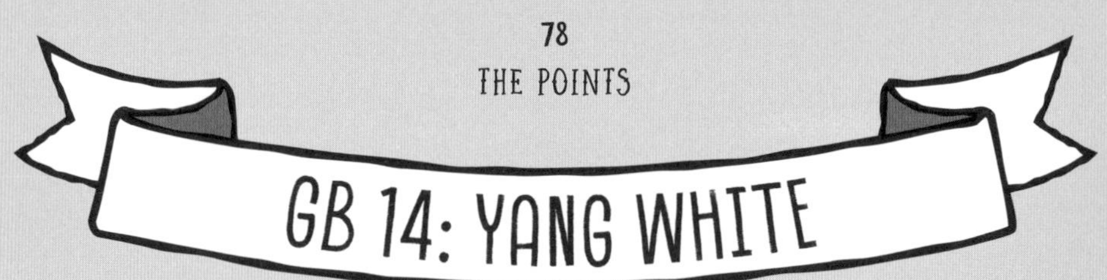

GB 14: YANG WHITE

Located on the forehead, directly above the pupil, 1 cun above the midpoint of the eyebrow.

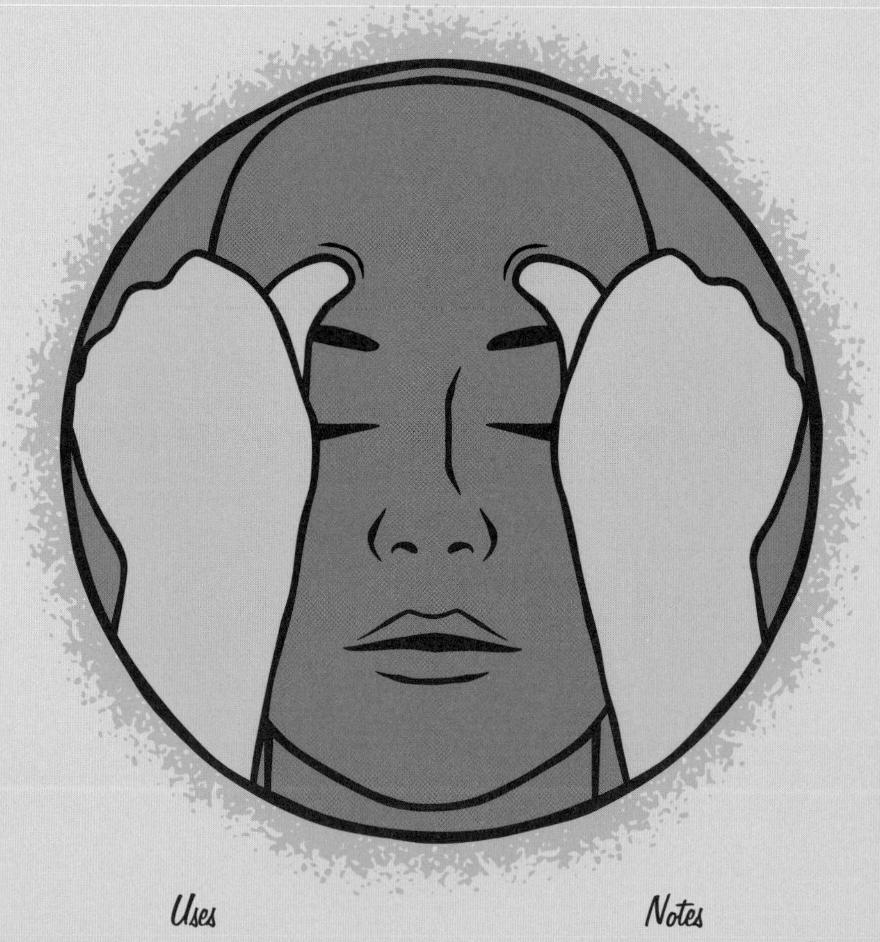

Uses

Used for forehead pains, frontal and temporal headaches, blurry vision, and eye pain.

Notes

To increase effect, rotate eyes with closed lids while pressing the point.

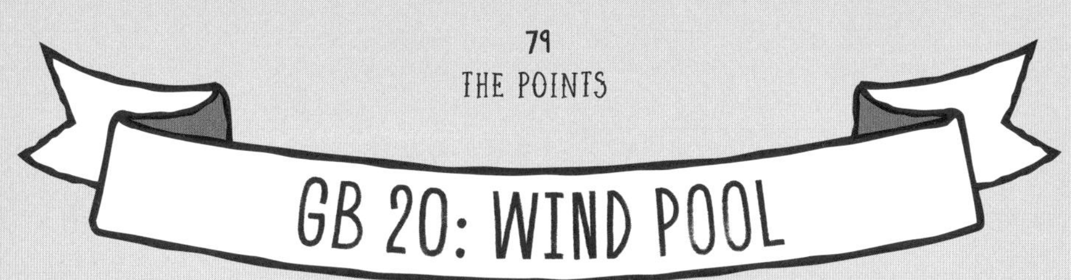

GB 20: WIND POOL

Located on the nape of the neck, in a depression roughly four finger's width from the spine.

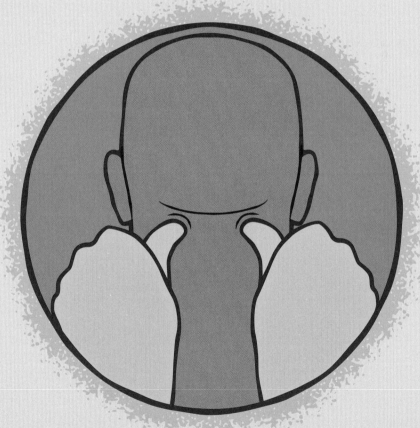

Uses

Used for issues related to the common cold, nasal congestion, headache, redness, swelling and pain of the eye, neck pain, limitation of the shoulder, dizziness, and vertigo.

Notes

GB 20 is a very useful point when treating any issues related to head, neck, and shoulder pain.

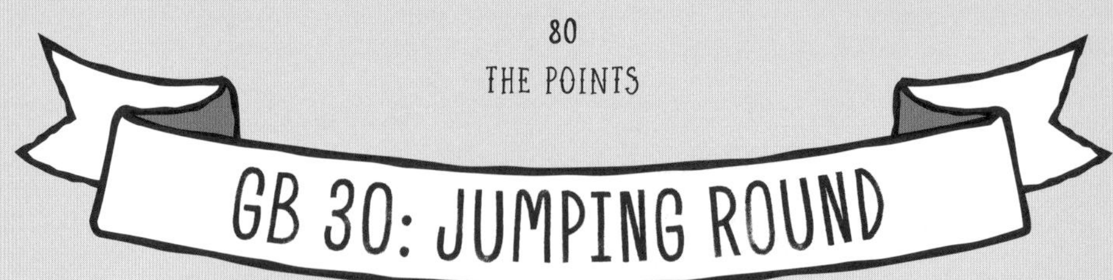

GB 30: JUMPING ROUND

While lying on the side with a flexed hip and knee, this point can be found on the outside of the buttocks, two-thirds of the distance between the greater trochanter and the coccyx.

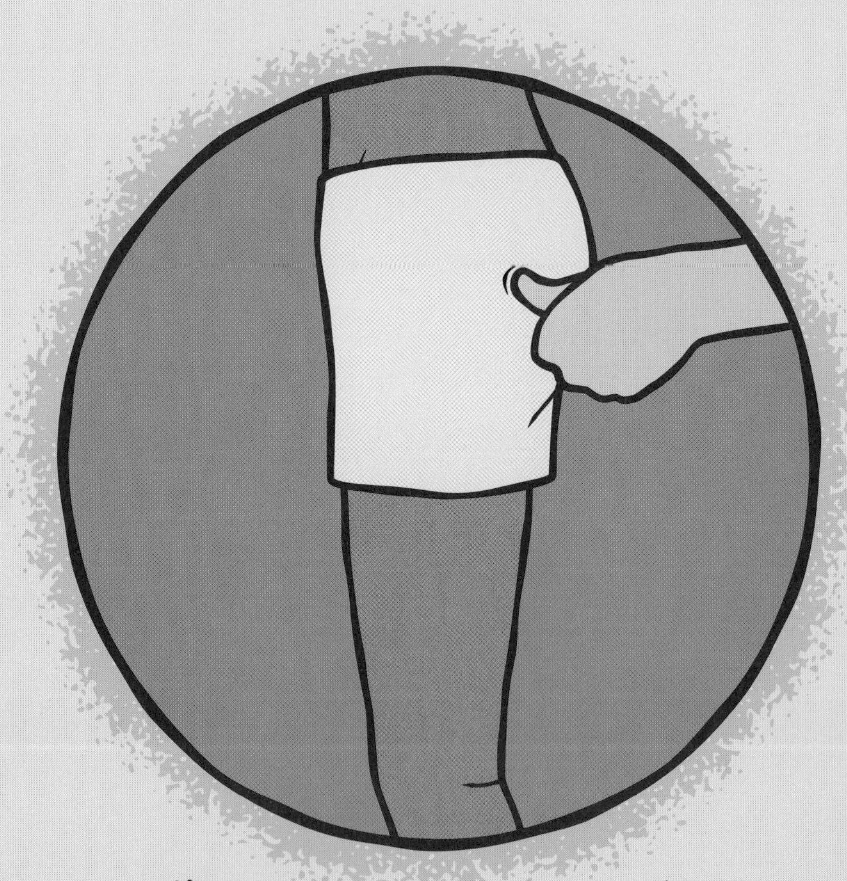

Uses

Commonly used point for lower back, hip, and leg issues.

Notes

Very useful point for pain related to sciatica and piriformis syndrome.

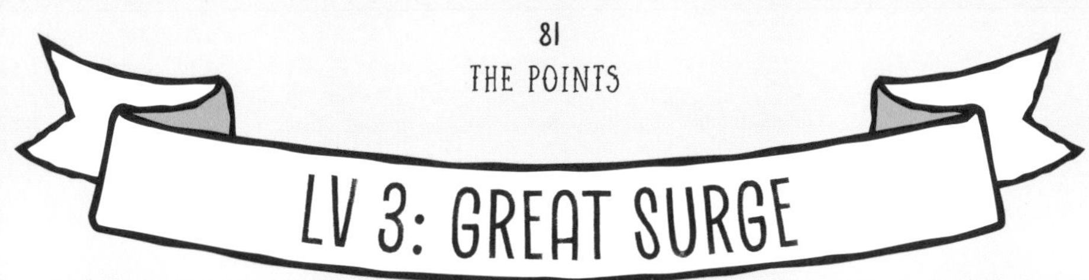

LV 3: GREAT SURGE

Found in a depression on the dorsum of the foot distal to the junctions of the first and second metatarsal bones.

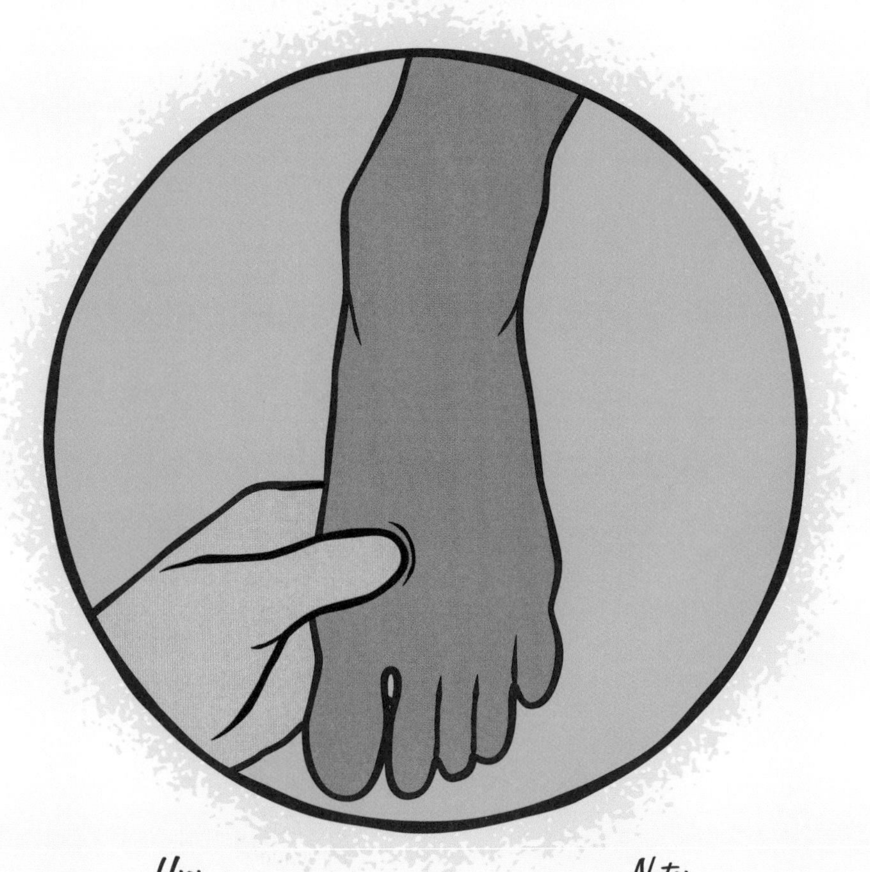

Uses

Used for blurry vision, swollen, painful eyes, dysmennorrhea, amenorrhea, PMS, breast tenderness, pain and swelling in the genitals, hernia, and digestive issues such as nausea, vomiting, constipation, and diarrhea.

Notes

One of the most commonly used points, LV 3 is often used with LI 4 (see page 43) to move qi and blood throughout the body.

LV 13: CAMPHORWOOD GATE

Located on the lateral side of the abdomen, below the free end of the eleventh floating rib.

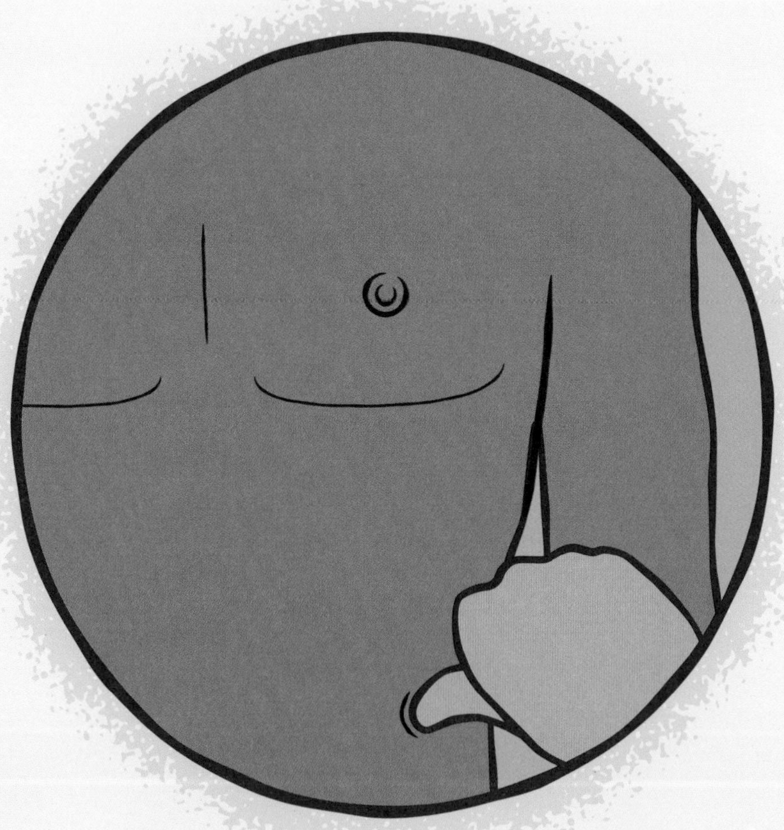

Uses

Used for distention in the abdomen, diarrhea with undigested food, vomiting, constipation, and bloating.

Notes

Known to help with spleen deficiency (see page 21).

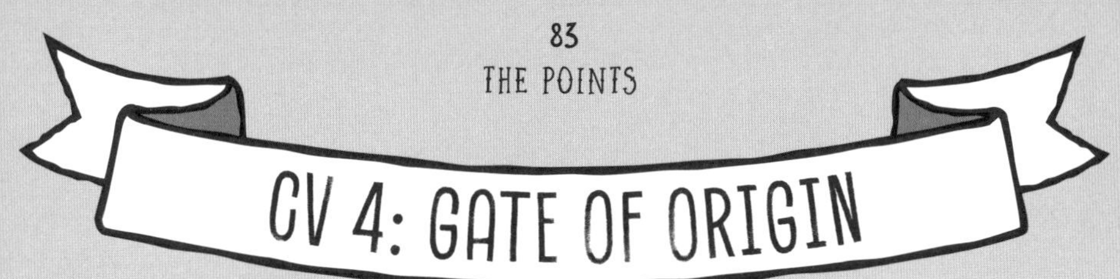

CV 4: GATE OF ORIGIN

Located on the abdomen, 3 cun below the belly button.

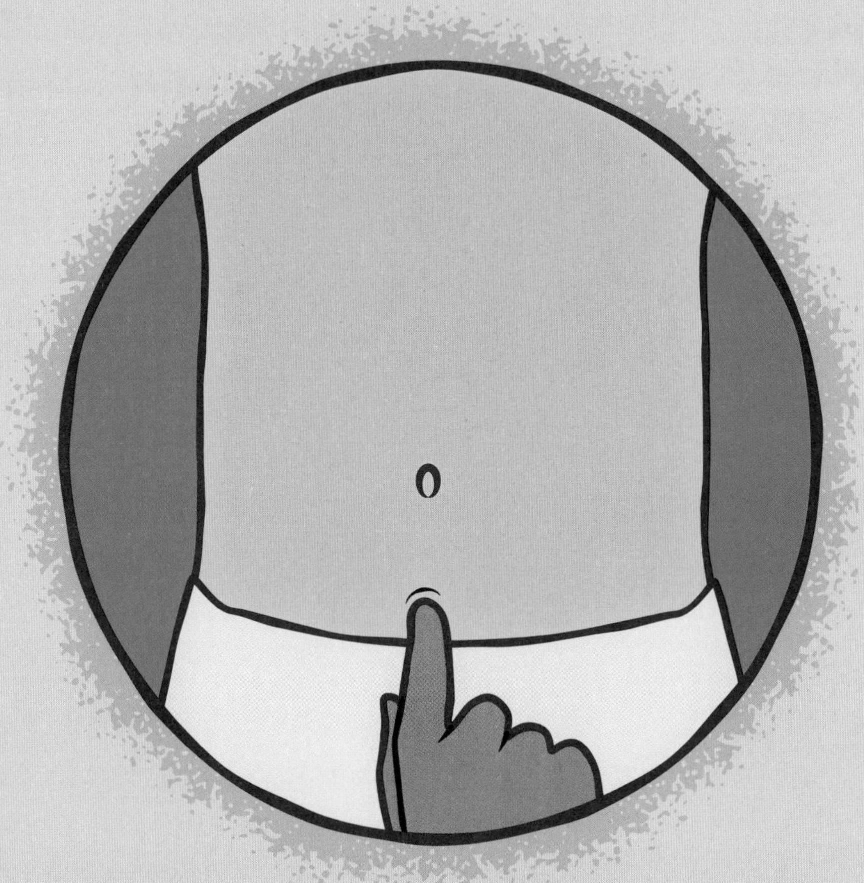

Uses

Commonly used for painful urination, impotence, irregular or painful menstruation, infertility, and hernia.

Notes

CV 4 is considered to be very useful for qi and blood deficiencies (see page 21). It is also an overall health maintenance point.

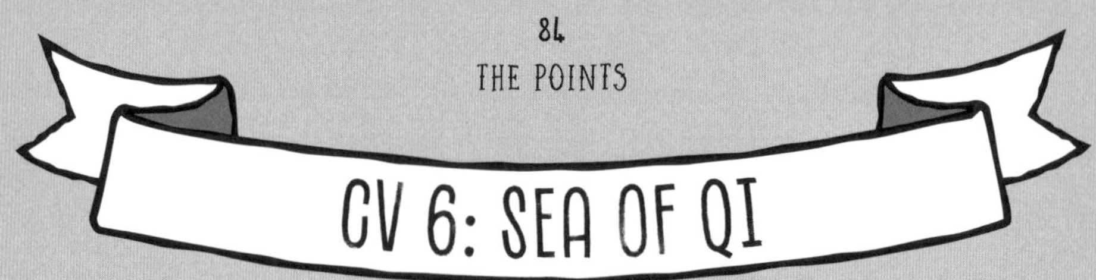

CV 6: SEA OF QI

Located on the abdomen, 1.5 cun below the belly button.

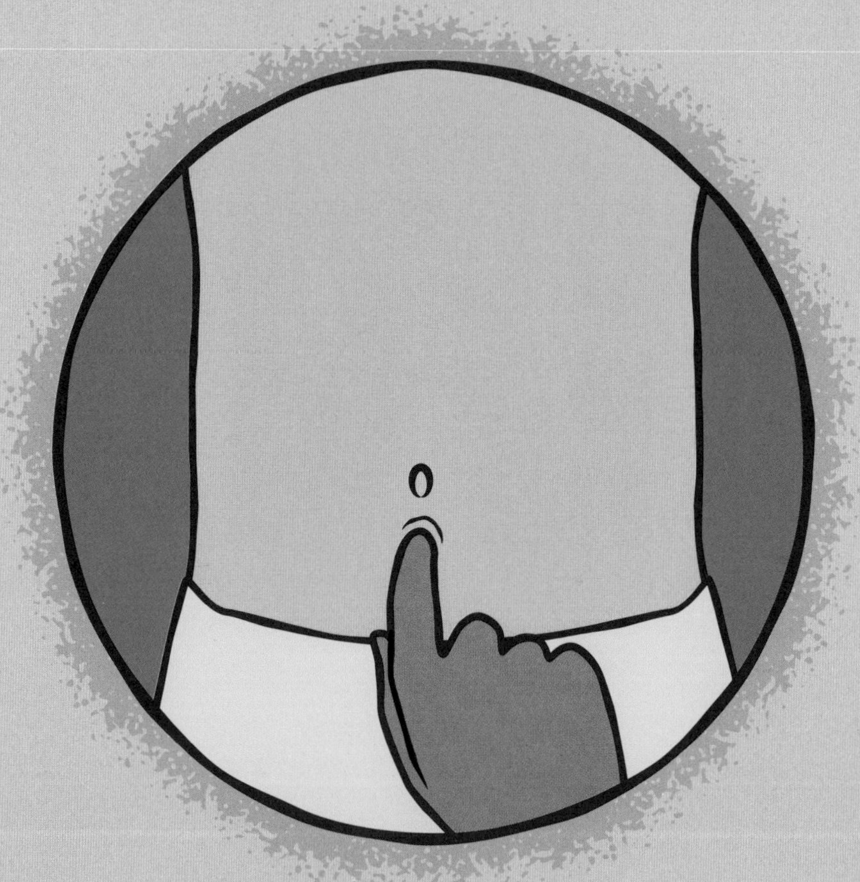

Uses

Commonly used for abdominal pain, diarrhea, and constipation.

Notes

CV 6 is considered to be the main point for rectum and uterine prolapses. Also known to maintain overall health.

CV 12: CENTRAL VENTER

Located on the abdomen, 4 cun above the belly button.

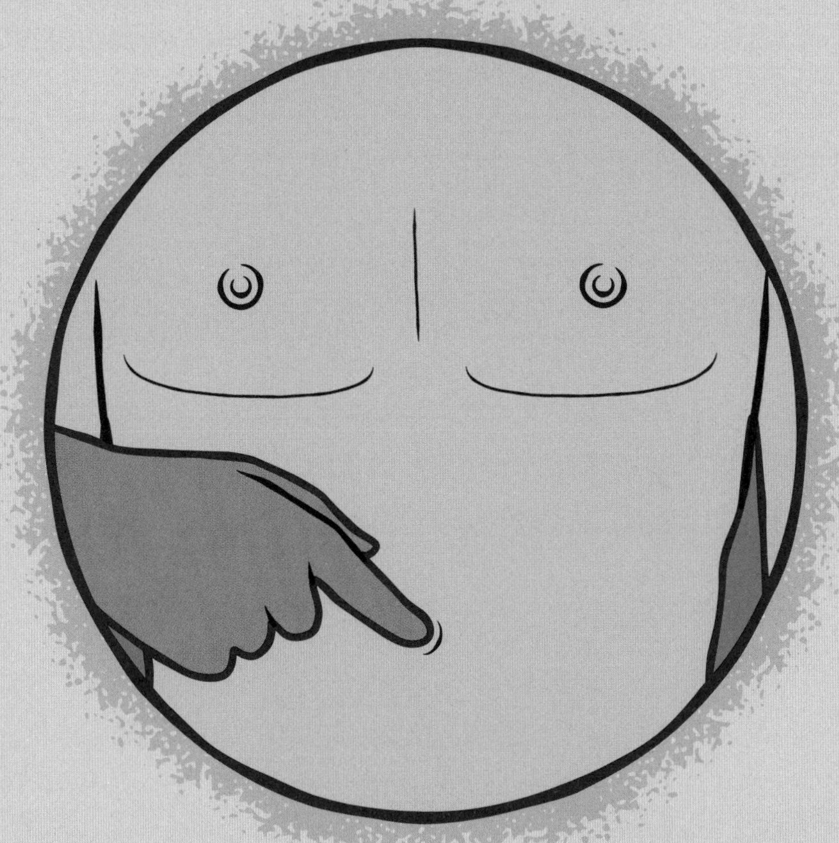

Uses

Commonly used for many digestive issues, such as bloating, acid reflux, nausea, diarrhea, and heartburn.

Notes

CV 12 is considered very useful for stress-induced digestive issues.

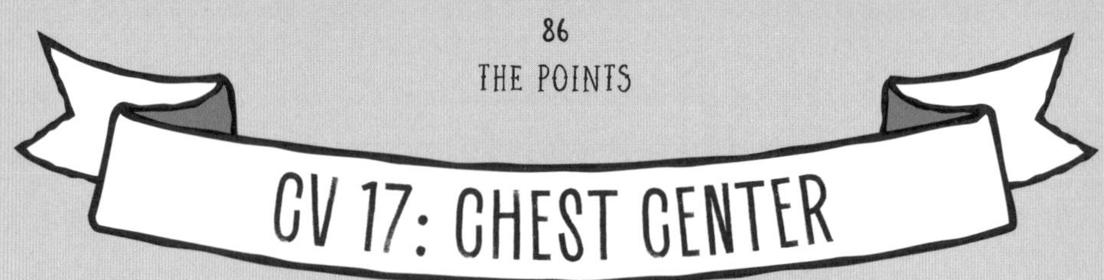

CV 17: CHEST CENTER

Located in the middle of the chest, at the level of the fourth intercostal space, midway between the nipples.

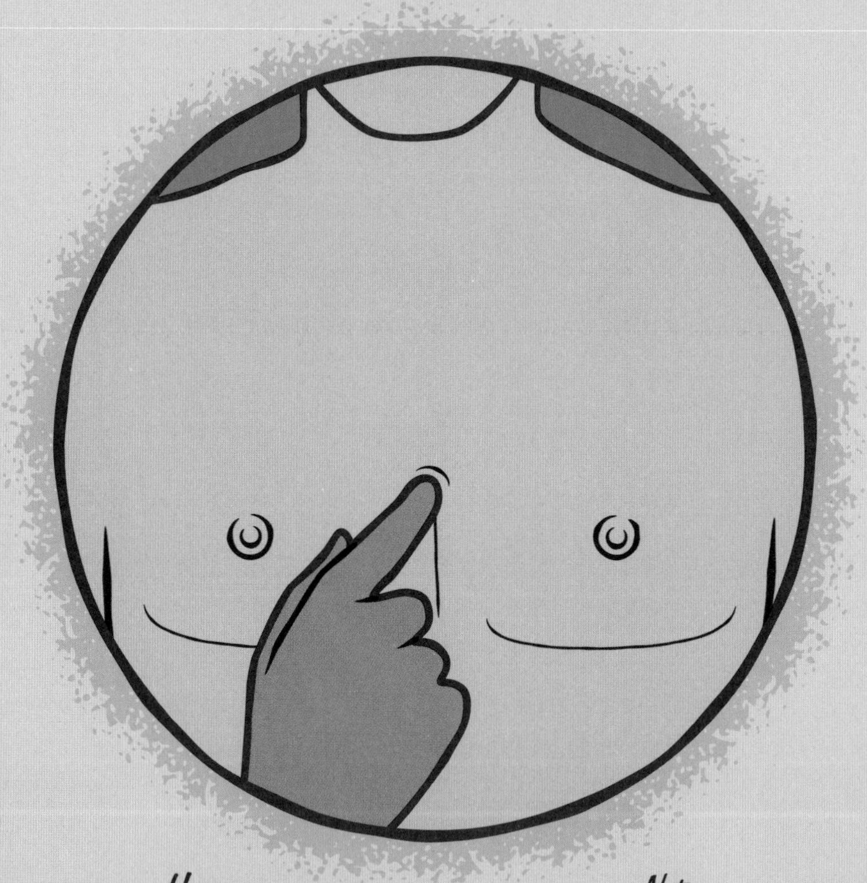

Uses

Commonly used for coughing, asthma, general pain in the chest, palpitations, insufficient lactation, and hiccups.

Notes

CV 17 is useful for helping to descend upperward-flowing, rebellious qi (burping, indigestion).

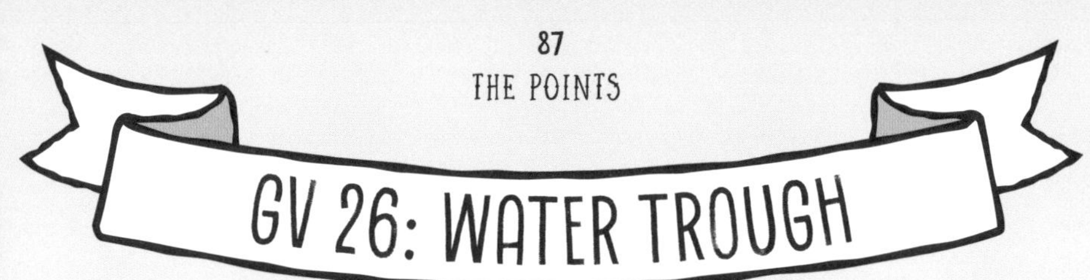

GV 26: WATER TROUGH

Located on the face, in the middle of the depression between the upper lip and the nose.

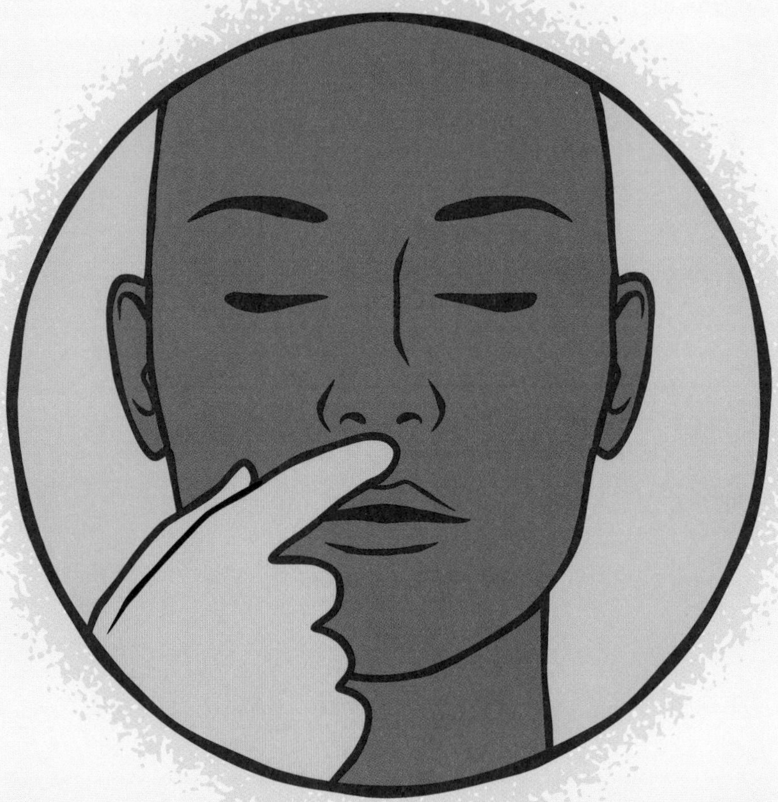

Uses

Commonly used to revive an unconscious person. GV 26 is also used for heatstroke, acute lumbar pain, and swelling of the face.

Notes

One of the main points for fainting and restoring consciousness. Pressed with a fingernail, GV 26 is said to help people awaken from passing out.

4 TREATMENT PLANS

A doctor who treats disease after it has happened is a mediocre doctor. A doctor who treats disease before it happens is a superior docotr.

YELLOW EMPEROR

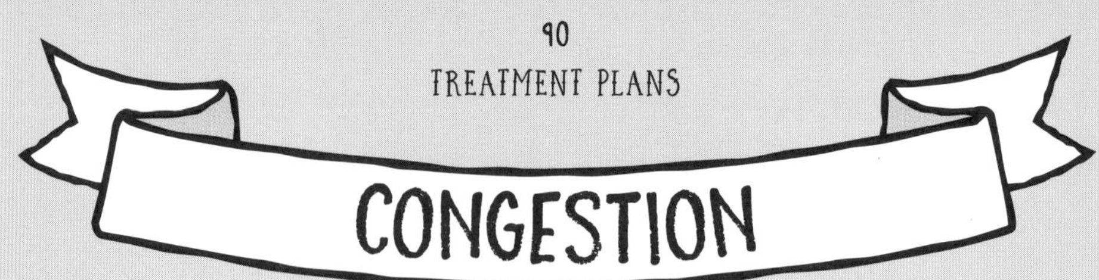

CONGESTION

Congestion is the experience of both inflammation in the nasal passages as well as a buildup of mucus as the body attempts to clear out the infection-causing agent. In cases of a common cold, a virus attaches to either the nose or throat after white blood cells fail to defend against the invasion. Often your body will feel weak or tired due to resources being diverted to help restore balance.

Additional Tips

Making loose fists, gently wrap against the upper part of the chest from LU 1 to the outside of the sternum to help break up chest congestion.

Self-Care

- **Head and Face** routine (see page 118)
- Chest portion of **Chest and Abdomen** routine (see page 121)
- Warm foods and liquids to break up congestion
- Hot baths or showers
- Rest

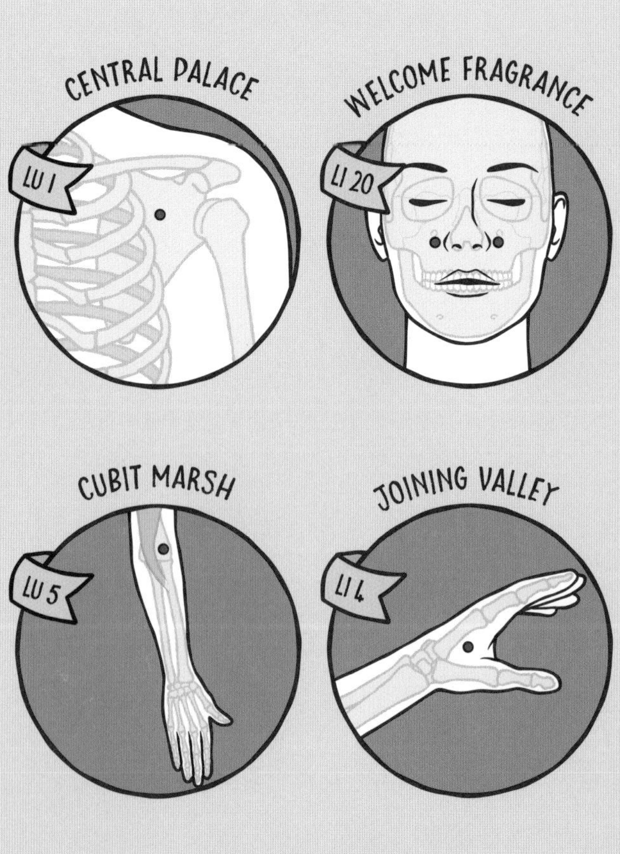

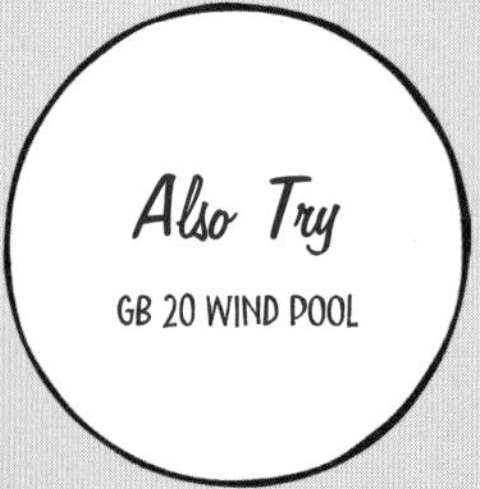

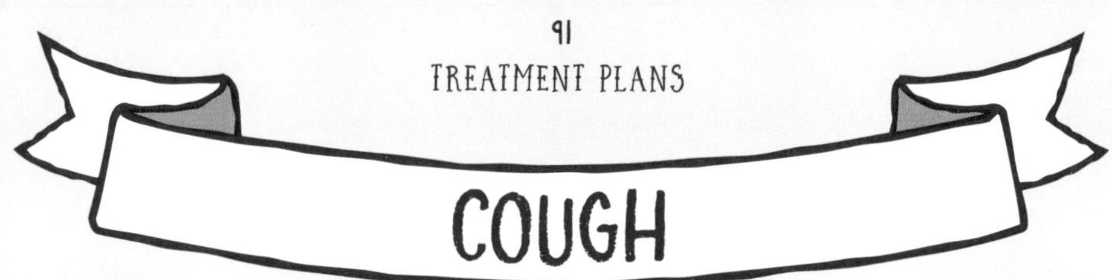

COUGH

Coughing is the body's mechanism for expectorating phlegm and debris from the upper respiratory system after a person has caught a cold. In Chinese Medicine, however, a cough is not just a symptom of getting sick. Rather, a cough may be due to either a deficiency or excess (see page 21), or to Cold, Heat, Damp, or Dry phenomena (see page 20), all of which can be diagnosed according to the quality of the phlegm produced.

Additional Tips

To invigorate and warm the points behind the lungs, try quick, horizontal, warming strokes back and forth with a flat palm across UB 12 and UB 13.

Self-Care

- **Head and Face** routine (see page 118)
- Chest portion of **Chest and Abdomen** routine (see page 121)
- Warm foods and liquids to break up congestion
- Hot baths or showers
- Rest

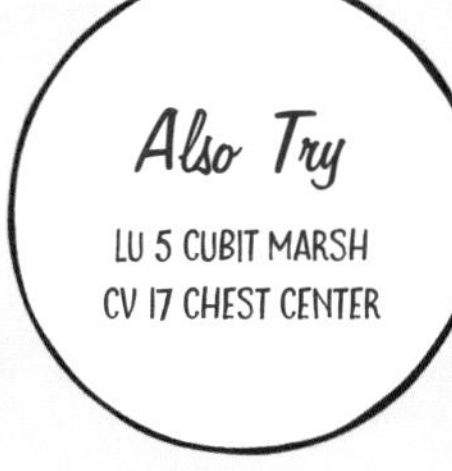

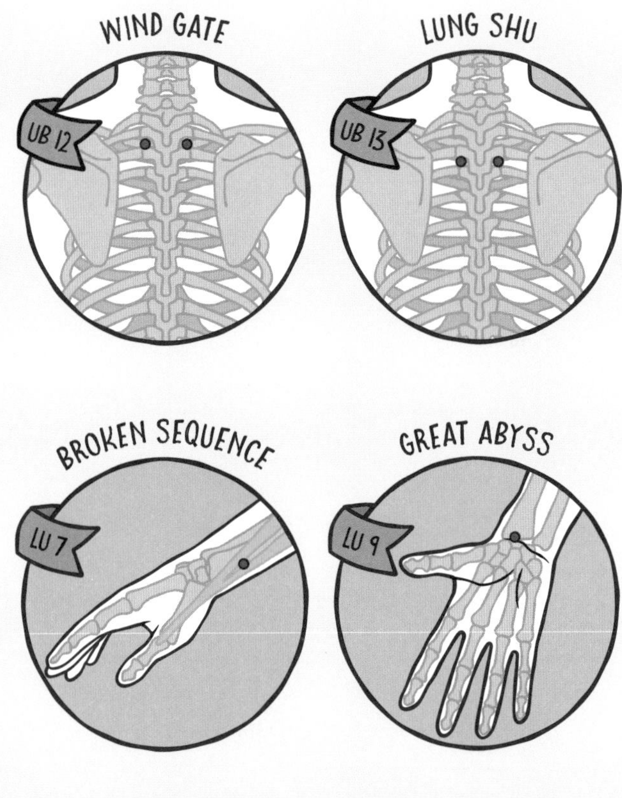

SORE THROAT

A sore throat is any pain, discomfort, or irritation in the throat, often experienced upon swallowing. From a TCM (Traditional Chinese Medicine) perspective, sore throats are often due to excess Heat (see page 20) present in the upper respiratory tract. Cooling the lungs and clearing Heat is therefore key to any treatment for sore throat.

Additional Tips

Since both points can often be tender, applying rou fa, or round rubbing (see page 30), to these points can be very soothing.

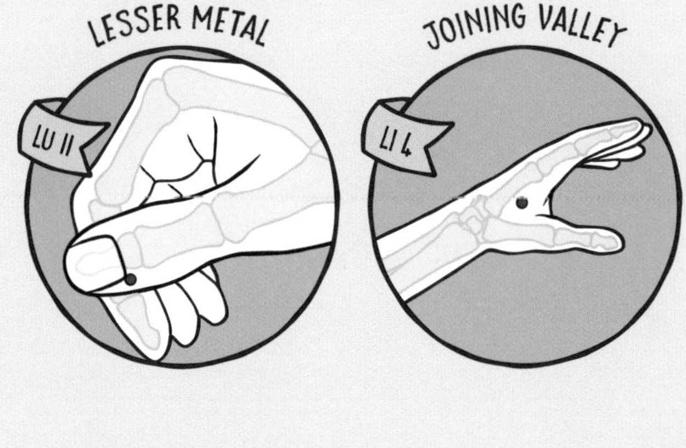

Self-Care

- **Head and Face** routine (see page 118)
- Chest portion of **Chest and Abdomen** routine (see page 121)
- Honey
- Rest

Also Try

KD 3 GREAT RAVINE

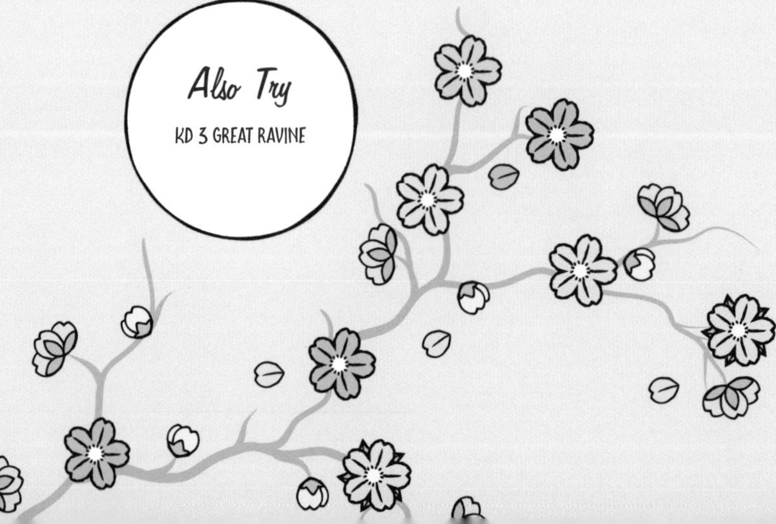

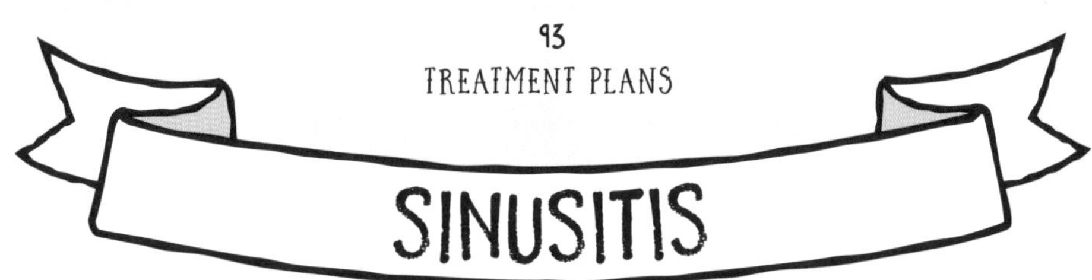

SINUSITIS

As its name suggests, sinusitis is inflammation of the sinuses, often caused by a buildup of mucus and phlegm, which create an environment ripe for infection.

Additional Tips

Even though it may be difficult, try to take long deep inhales through the nose while pressing or rubbing the points.

Self-Care

- **Head and Face** routine (see page 118)
- Chest portion of **Chest and Abdomen** routine (see page 121)
- Avoid phlegm-causing foods and drinks such as dairy products
- Warm foods and liquids to break up congestion
- Hot baths or showers
- Inhaling steam from a bowl with eucalyptus essential oil

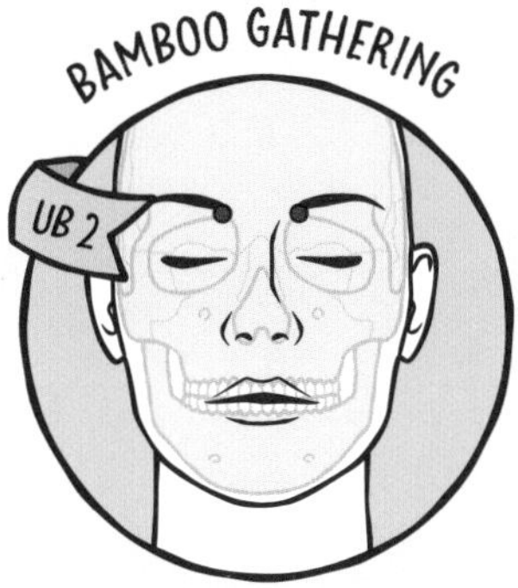

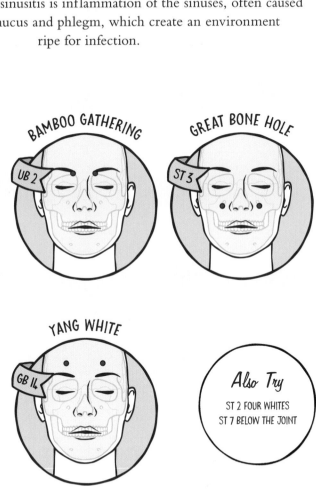

BAMBOO GATHERING
UB 2

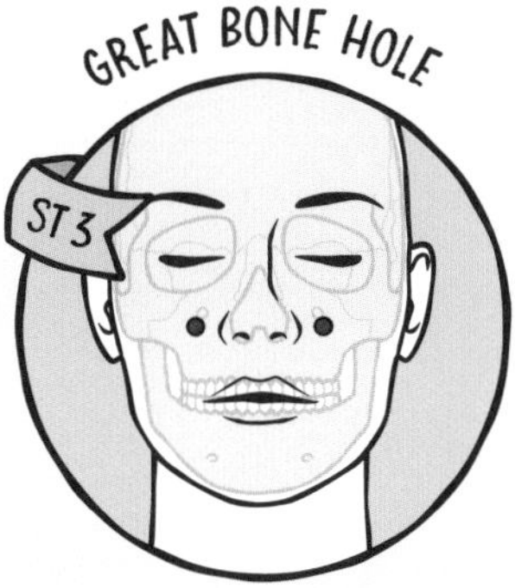

GREAT BONE HOLE
ST 3

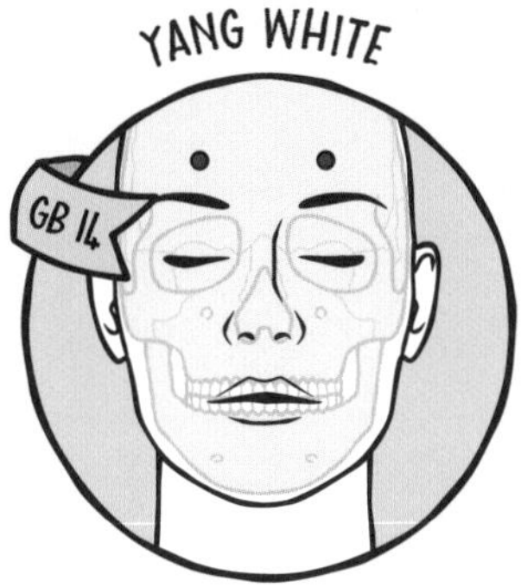

YANG WHITE
GB 14

Also Try

ST 2 FOUR WHITES
ST 7 BELOW THE JOINT

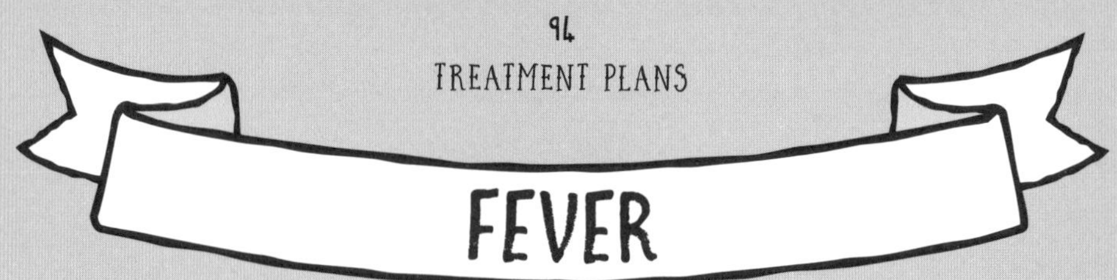

FEVER

A fever is the body's natural and healthy response to fighting off bacteria that thrive at the normal body temperature. While most fevers are beneficial, and are not cause for alarm, many people crave some cooling relief from the increase in body temperature.

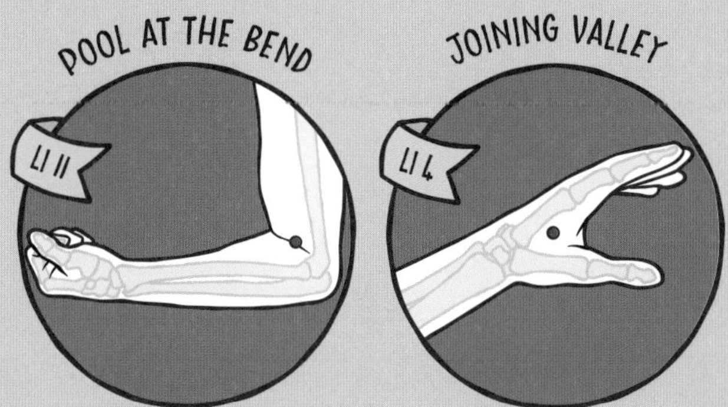

Additional Tips

Before you rush to the medicine chest to suppress your fever, know that temperatures below 103°F (39°C) in adults, while uncomfortable, are still considered safe and beneficial. In fact, by reducing a fever too quickly, you run the risk of prolonging the infection.

Self-Care

- Cool towel on forehead
- Rest

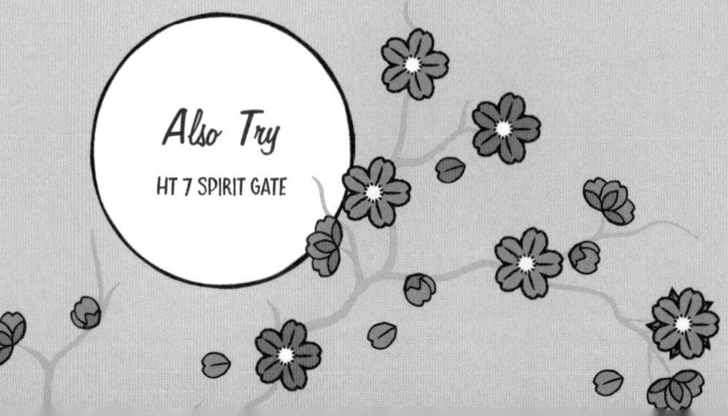

HEADACHES

An episodic tension headache may be described as a mild to moderate, constant, band-like pain, tightness, or pressure around the forehead or the back of the head and neck.

Additional Tips

Using the pads of the fingers, gently massage any particular areas of tension around the head to help soothe muscles.

Self-Care

- **Head and Face** routine (see page 118)
- **Neck and Shoulders** routine (see page 119)

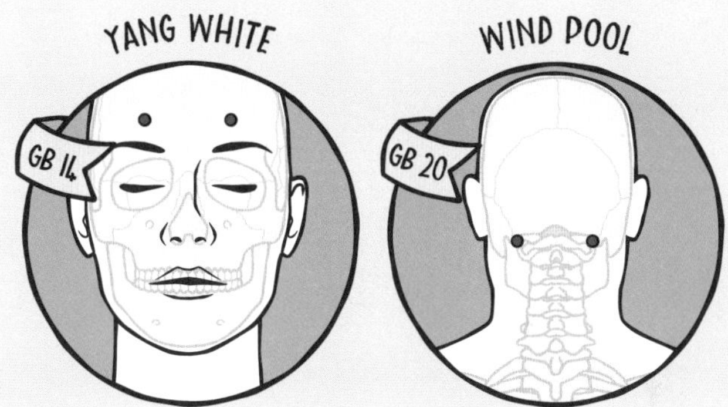

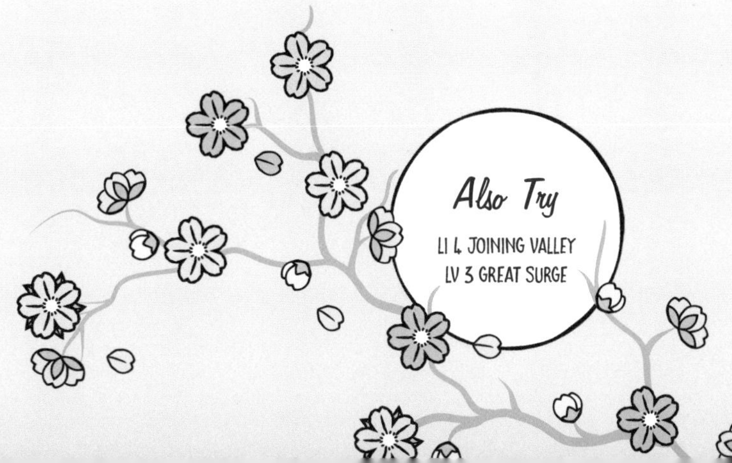

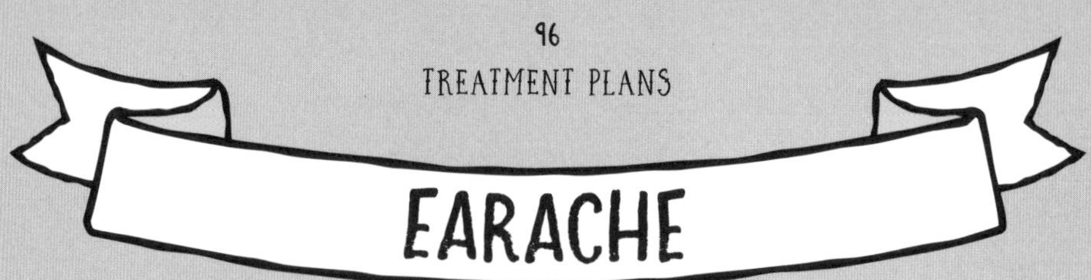

EARACHE

From a TCM (Traditional Chinese Medicine) perspective, an earache is often the result of Wind or Wind-Heat (see page 20) invading the ear, presenting as not only pain in the ear canal, but also sometimes a "stuffed" feeling in the ear, as well as corresponding head and body aches. Acupressure treatments will usually involve points that help to clear Wind and Wind-Heat.

Additional Tips

Massaging these points using gentle circular motions can help to relieve pain in the ear.

Self-Care

- **Head and Face** routine (see page 118)
- **Neck and Shoulders** routine (see page 119)
- Ear candles
- Lying down on alternating sides to both expose and drain the ear

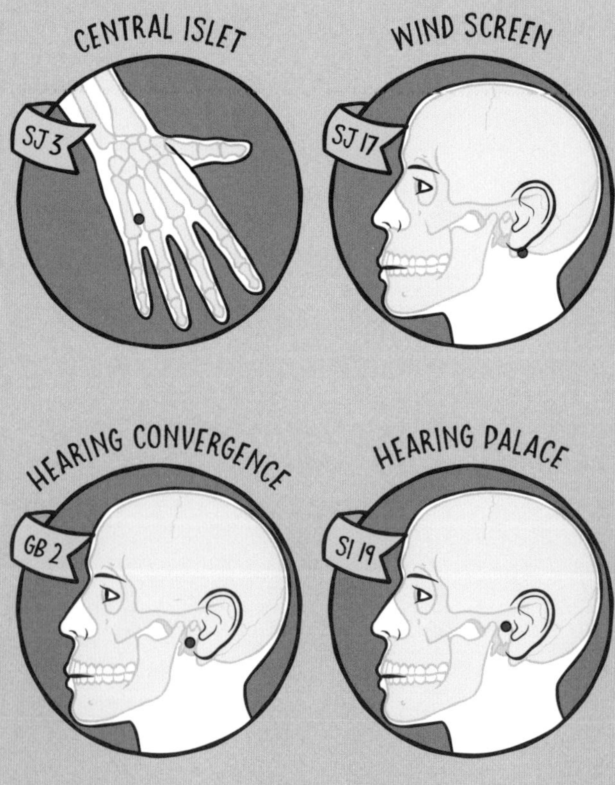

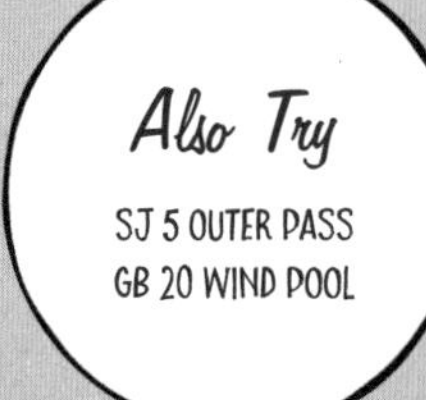

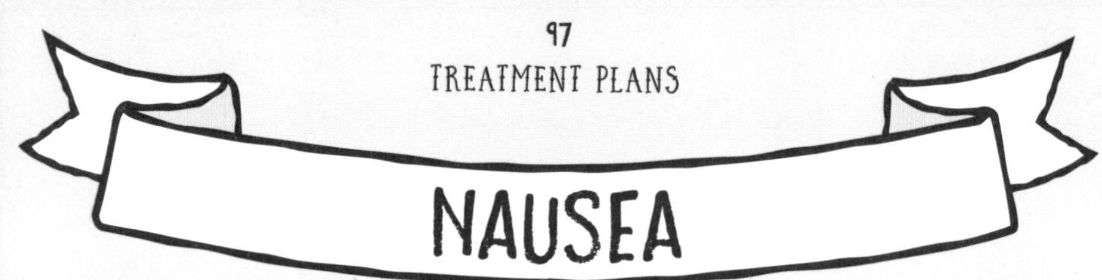

NAUSEA

Nausea, the experience of uneasiness or potential regurgitation in the stomach, can be caused by many factors, including motion sickness, overeating, illness, medications, etc. From a TCM (Traditional Chinese Medicine) perspective, nausea is often understood as unsettled qi in the stomach, or heavy, damp qi related to overeating.

Additional Tips

Slow, warming, circular strokes with a flat palm on the abdomen in a clockwise fashion can be helpful for soothing nausea.

Self-Care

- **Lower Back** routine (see page 122)
- Abdomen portion of **Chest and Abdomen** routine (see page 121)
- Warm foods and liquids to break up congestion
- Hot baths or showers
- Rest

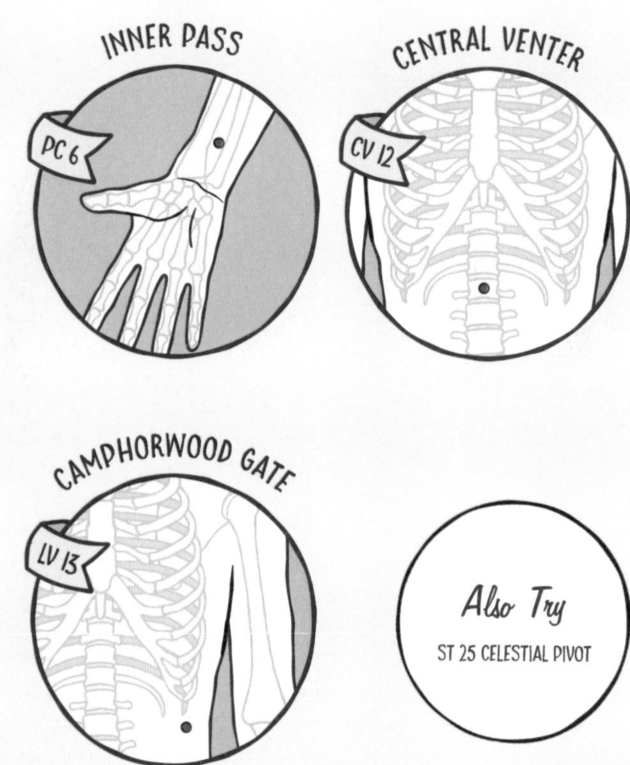

INDIGESTION

Indigestion has to do with pain or discomfort in the stomach associated with difficulty in digesting food. Symptoms include burning in the stomach or upper abdomen, abdominal pain, bloating (full feeling), belching and gas, nausea and vomiting, acidic taste, and growling stomach.

Additional Tips

Slowly warm the abdomen with a flat palm by making circles clockwise.

Self-Care

- **Head and Face** routine (see page 118)
- Abdomen portion of **Chest and Abdomen** routine (see page 121)

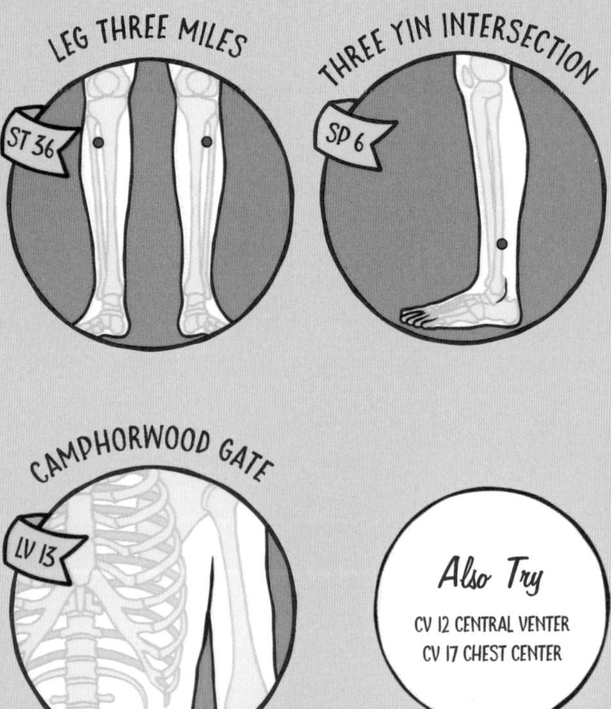

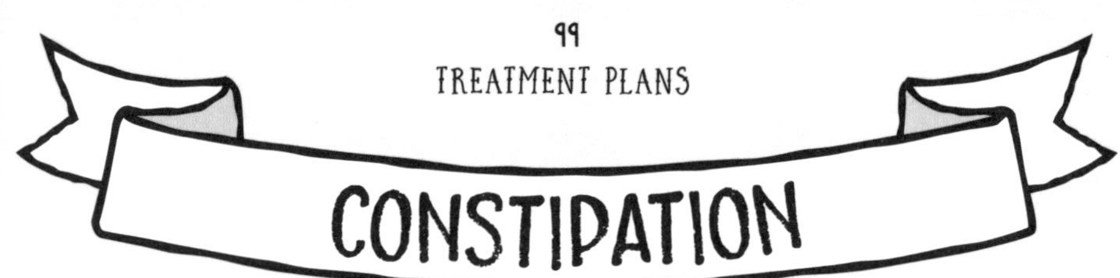

CONSTIPATION

Constipation is a condition in which there is difficulty emptying the bowels. Symptoms may include few and/or difficult bowel movements, hard or small stools, a sense that everything didn't come out, abdominal pain, and/or a swollen abdomen.

Additional Tips

Assisted hip rotations, as well as bringing the knees to the chest while lying on one's back or squatting, can help massage the abdomen and promote elimination.

Self-Care

- **Lower Back** routine (see page 122)
- Abdomen portion of **Chest and Abdomen** routine (see page 121)

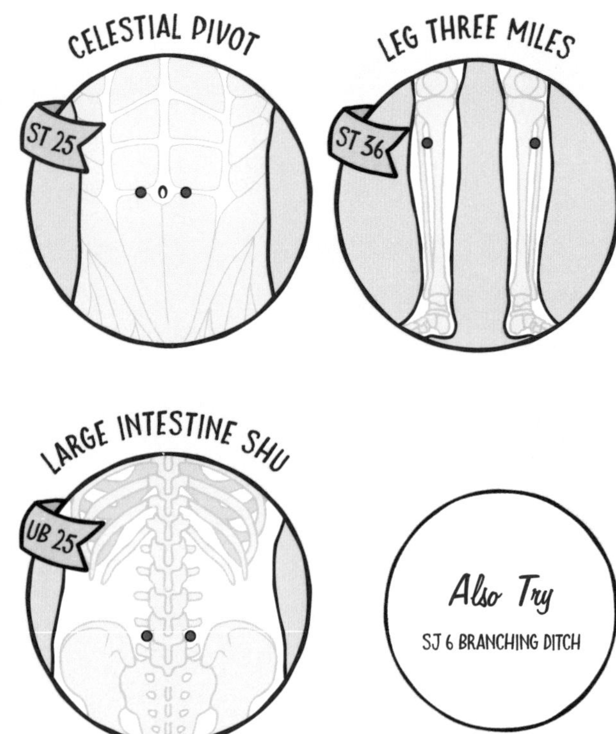

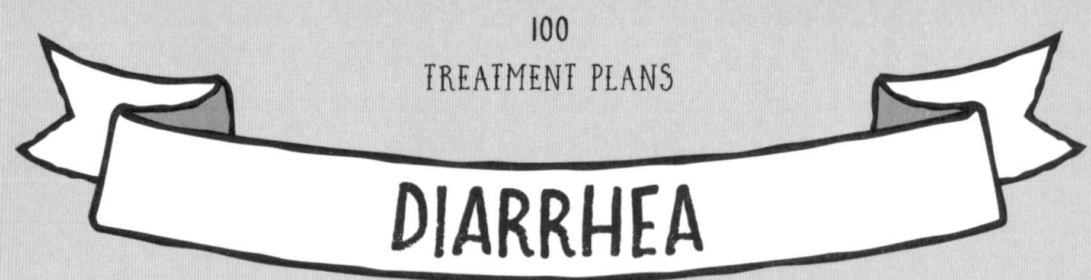

DIARRHEA

Diarrhea is known as looseness in the stool, characterized in the West usually as the body's malabsorption of fluid. This can be due to many factors, including diet, emotional issues, or bacterial infections. TCM (Traditional Chinese Medicine) diagnoses will often point to either a Cold, Damp-Heat, or Damp condition (see page 20) as the root cause.

Additional Tips

One should not be quick to halt diarrhea unless there is a danger of dehydration, or if a serious underlying condition is thought to be the cause. Like a fever, diarrhea can be a natural and healthy response, helping to rid the body of irritating agents.

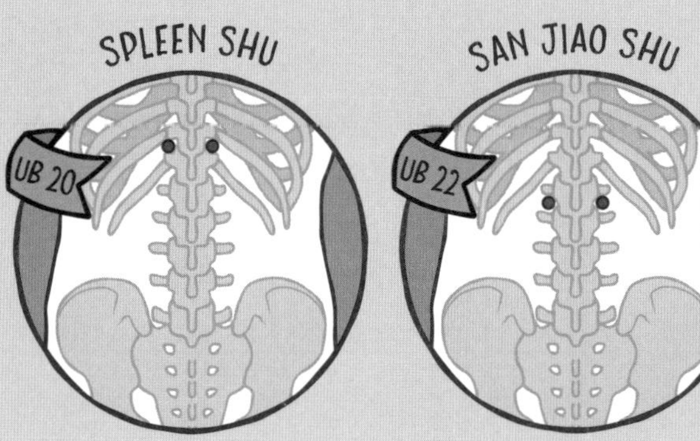

Self-Care

- Abdomen portion of **Chest and Abdomen** routine (see page 121)

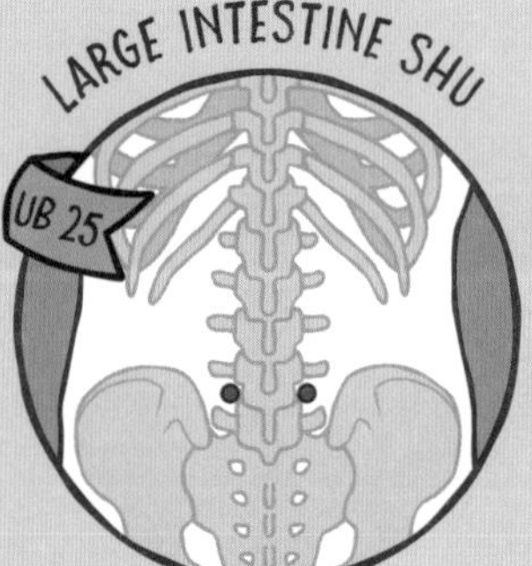

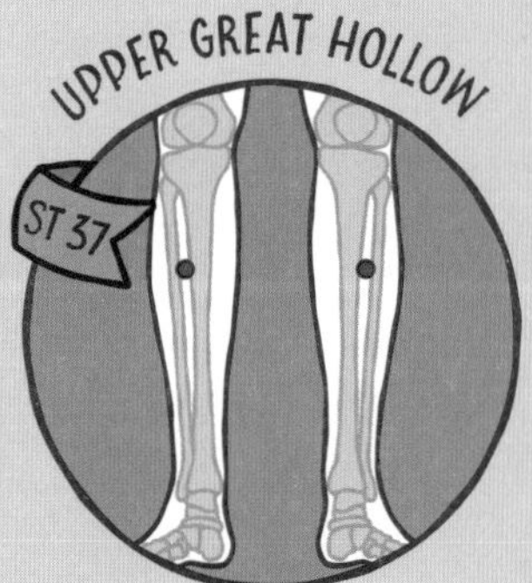

Also Try

SP 9 YIN MOUND SPRING

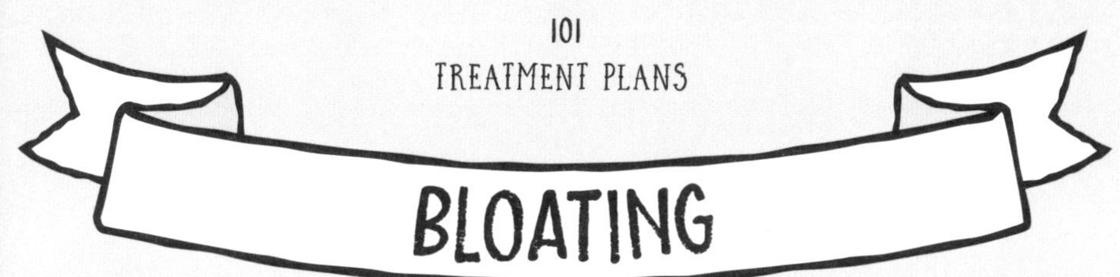

BLOATING

Bloating is the experience of a buildup of gas in the abdomen, causing distention and a feeling of tightness and pain. Relief is often found from expelling gas from the mouth or anus. Traditional Chinese Medicine considers bloating to be the result of Damp-Heat (see page 20) and/or a disharmony between the liver and spleen.

Additional Tips

Postural changes such as squatting or leaning with arms on a countertop, while swaying the back, can help relieve a buildup of gas.

Self-Care

- Abdomen portion of **Chest and Abdomen** routine (see page 121)
- Lying on back with knees into chest or squatting to relieve gas
- Avoid gas-causing foods and beverages

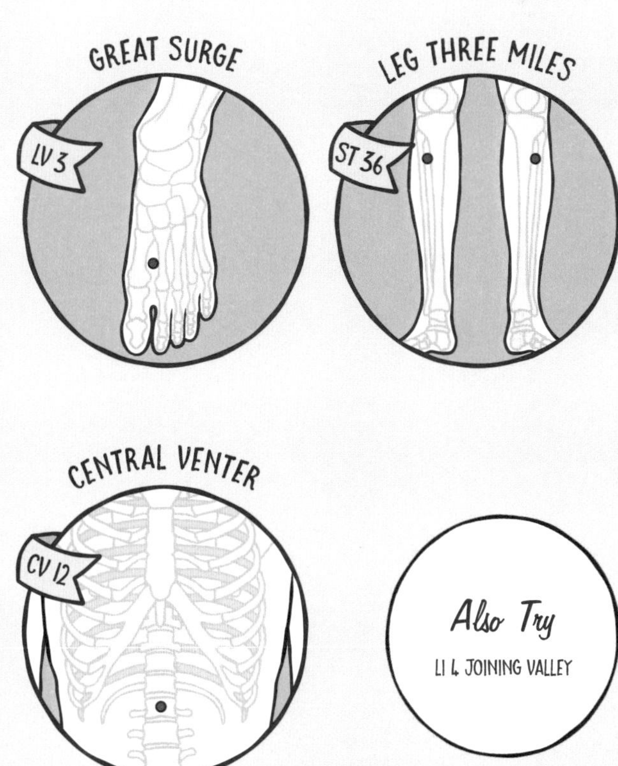

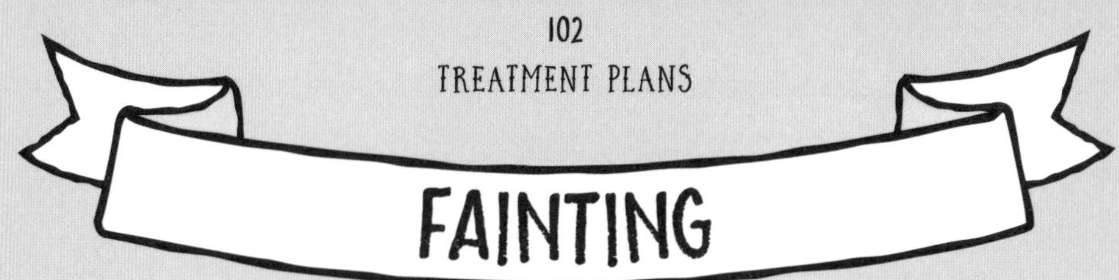

FAINTING

Fainting or "passing out" happens as a result of a momentary loss of consciousness due to a decrease in blood flow to the brain. In Chinese Medicine this would be considered a blood deficiency.

Additional Tips

Before anything else, make sure to loosen a person's clothing to relieve any constrictions around blood supply and air intake, and check for a pulse. Keep the legs elevated, and, if the person begins to vomit, turn them onto their side to prevent choking.

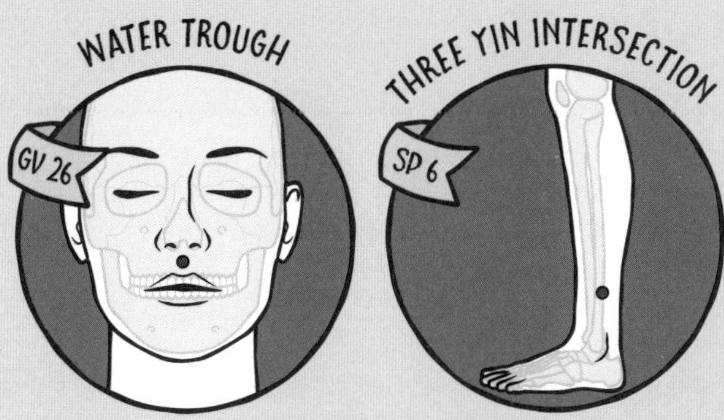

Self-Care

- See above

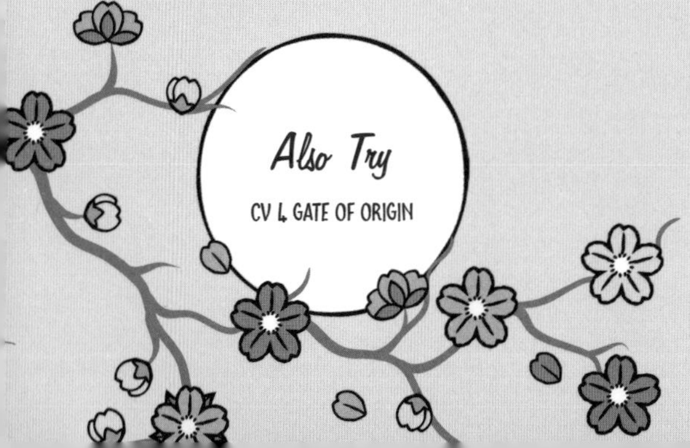

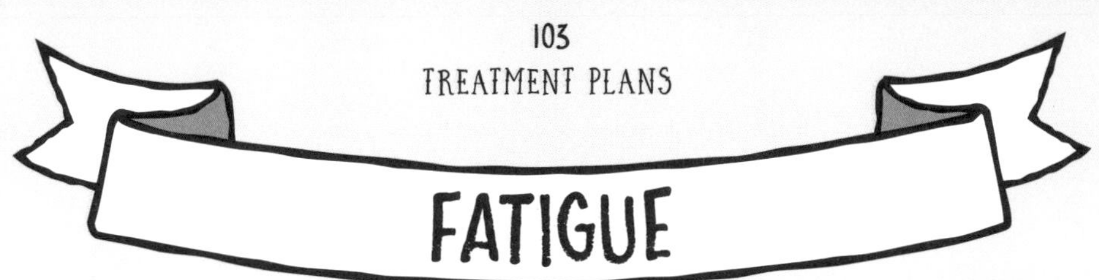

FATIGUE

Extreme tiredness typically results from mental or physical exertion or illness. Sufferers experience difficulty concentrating, anxiety, a gradual decrease in stamina, difficulty sleeping, and increased sensitivity to light. They also may skip social engagements once viewed as important to them.

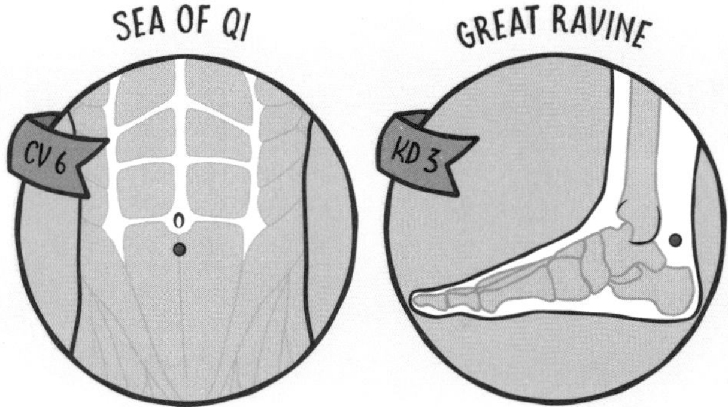

Additional Tips

Looking into better sleeping techniques, taking cold showers, and getting plenty of exercise and fresh air can all be helpful in combatting feelings of fatigue.

Self-Care

- Administer any routine (see pages 118–123) where person is feeling tension
- Exercise
- Cold showers

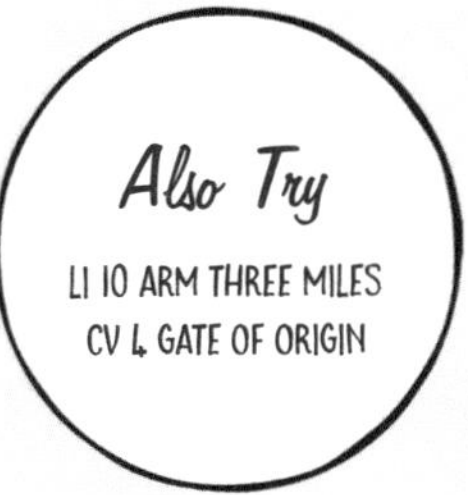

Also Try

LI 10 ARM THREE MILES
CV 4 GATE OF ORIGIN

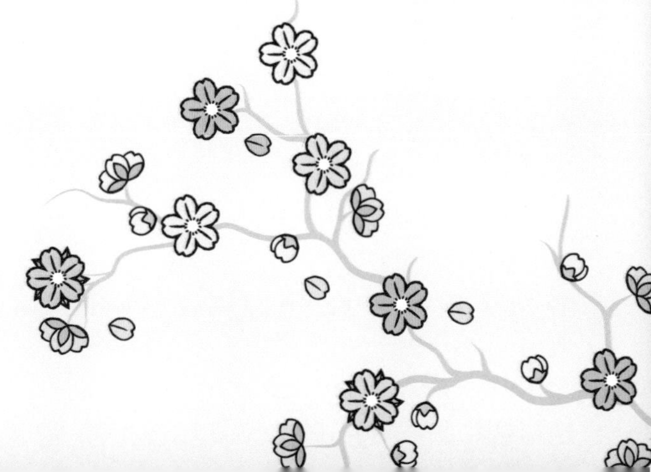

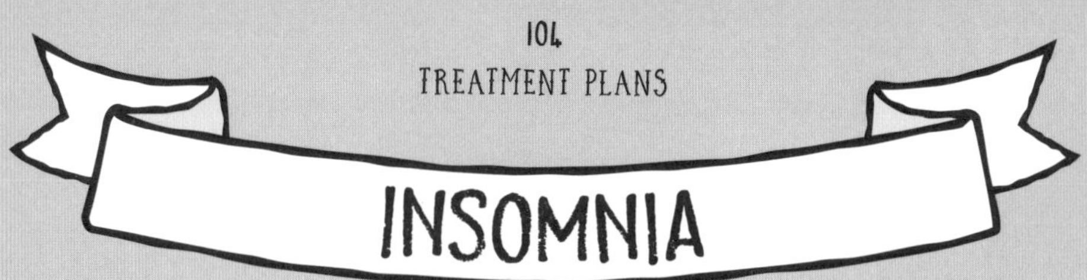

INSOMNIA

Insomnia is a sleep disorder characterized by difficulty falling and/or staying asleep, and may also include waking up too early in the morning, or feeling tired upon waking. Significant life stresses (job loss or change, death of a loved one, divorce, moving), illness, emotional or physical discomfort, environmental factors like noise, light, or extreme temperatures (hot or cold), and some medications (for example, those used to treat colds, allergies, depression, high blood pressure, and asthma) may all interfere with sleep.

Additional Tips

Working around the neck and head can be especially helpful for calming and settling the mind.

Self-Care

- **Head and Face** routine (see page 118)
- **Legs and Feet** routine (see page 123)

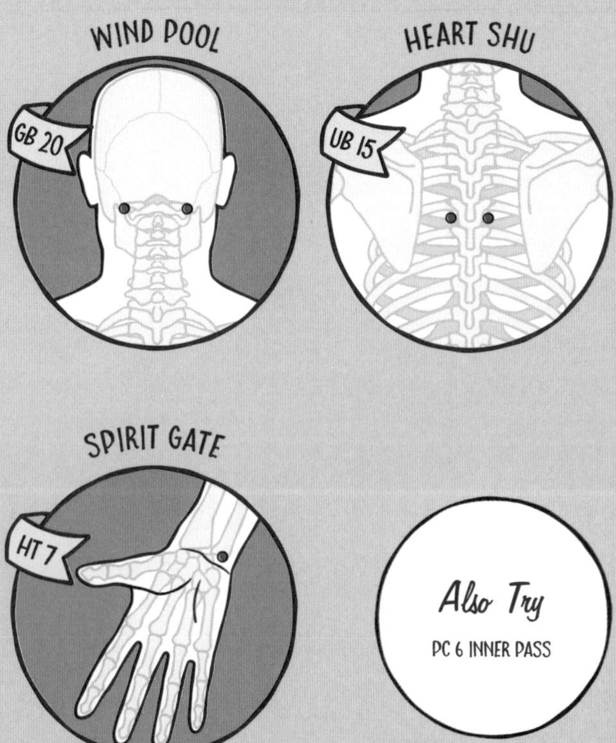

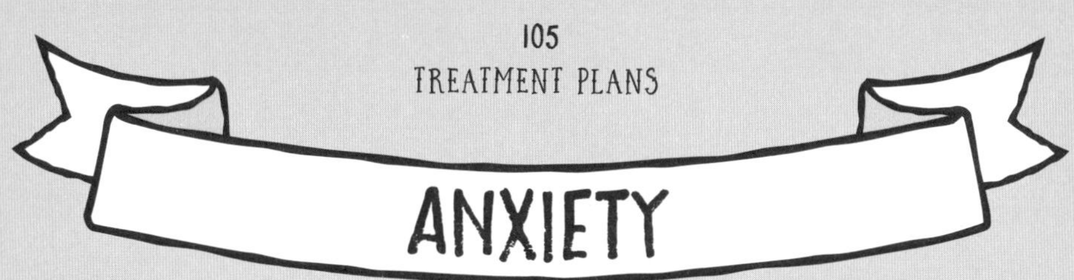

ANXIETY

Generally speaking, non-emergency anxiety is defined as a feeling of worry, nervousness, or unease, typically about an imminent event or something with an uncertain outcome.

Additional Tips

Moving the "feedback loop" of active energy "stuck" in the upper region of the body, specifically from solar plexus to head, into the lower body with massage can be very helpful.

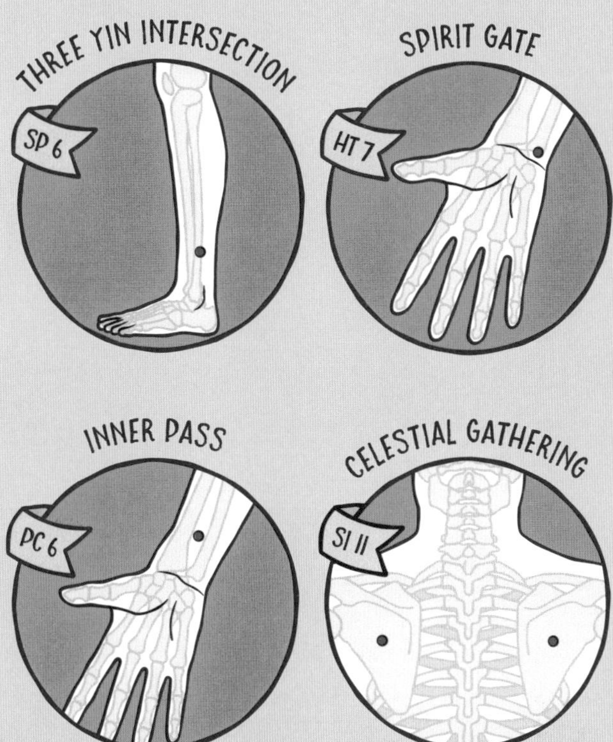

Self-Care

- **Neck and Shoulders** routine (see page 119)
- **Chest and Abdomen** routine (see page 121)
- **Legs and Feet** routine (see page 123)

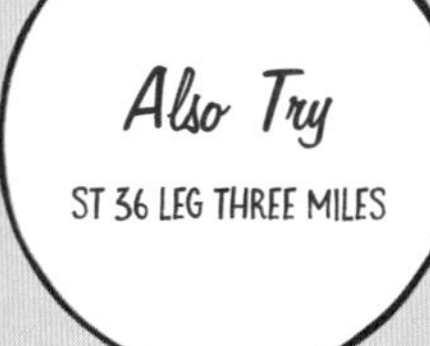

PAINFUL MENSTRUAL CRAMPS

Dysmenorrhea is the medical term for the painful cramps that may occur immediately before or during the menstrual period. Cramps usually begin one to two years after a woman starts getting her period. Pain is usually felt in the lower abdomen or back. They can be mild to severe. Common menstrual cramps often start shortly before or at the onset of the period and continue for one to three days. Scant or difficult menstrual flow may be associated with dysmenorrhea.

Additional Tips

Placing a hot water bottle and towel over the abdomen and lower back can help to reduce pain and discomfort.

Self-Care

- **Lower Back** routine (see page 122)

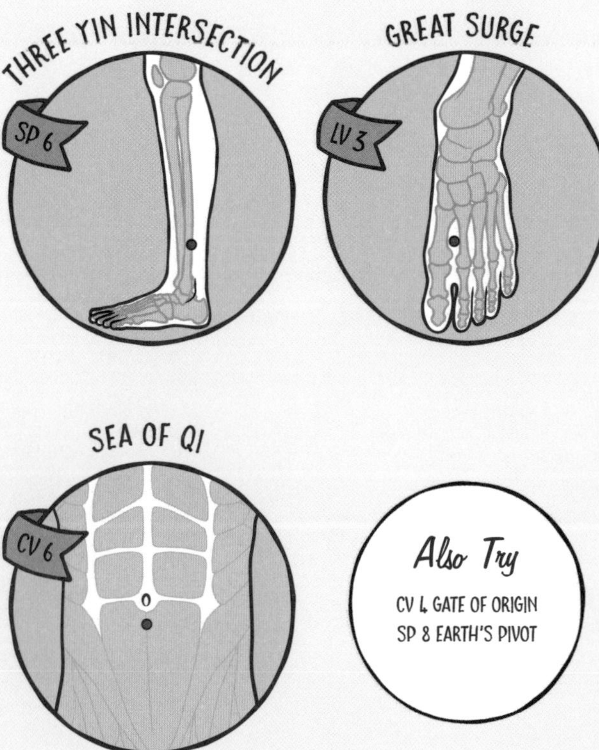

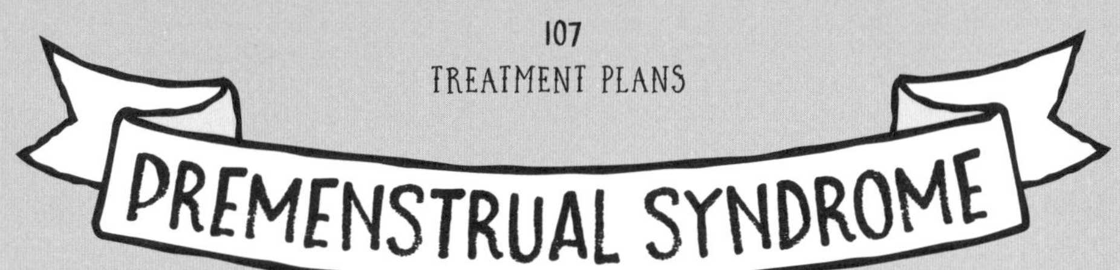

PREMENSTRUAL SYNDROME

The physical and emotional experiences that a woman may have a few days before the onset of her menstrual cycle, including tender breasts, bloating, cramps, mood swings, and headaches, are normal premenstrual symptoms. However, when they disrupt daily life, they are called premenstrual syndrome (PMS). Specific physiological symptoms include joint or muscle pain, headache, fatigue, weight gain related to fluid retention, abdominal bloating, breast tenderness, acne flare-ups, constipation, or diarrhea.

Additional Tips

Using any routines that apply to areas of specific stress in the body can be very helpful.

Self-Care

- **Neck and Shoulders** routine (see page 119)
- **Lower Back** routine (see page 122)

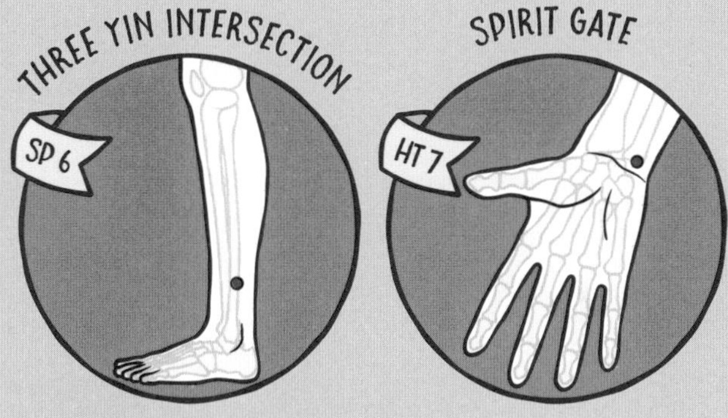

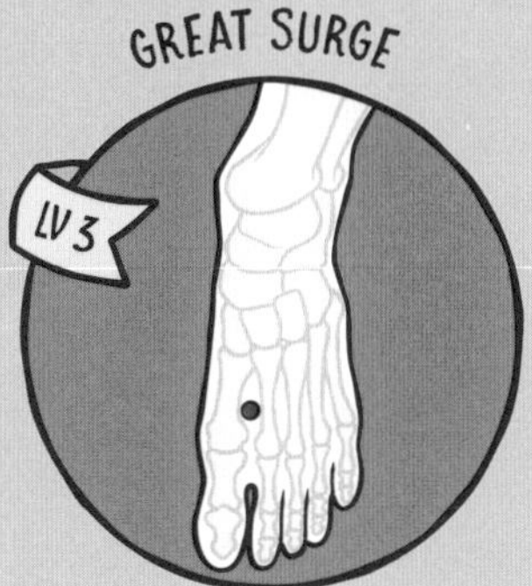

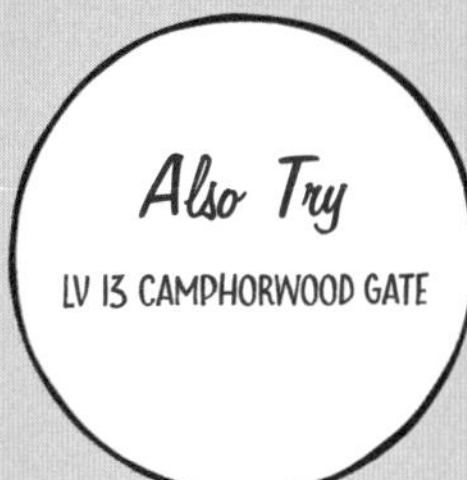

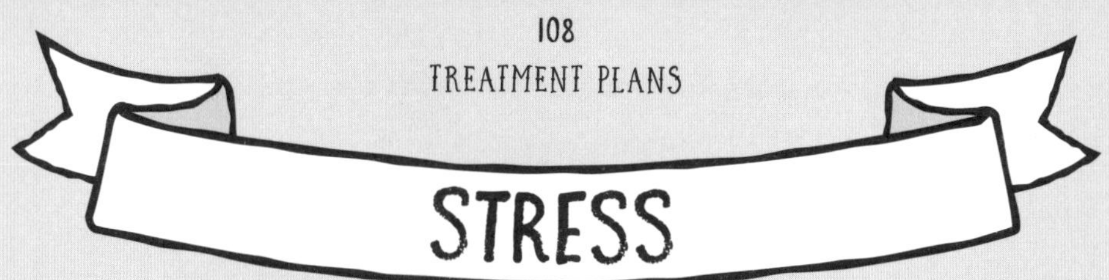

STRESS

Negative stress is the feeling we have when under pressure, while stressors are the things we respond to in our environment. Examples of stressors are noises, unpleasant people, a speeding car, or even going out on a first date.

Generally (but not always), the more stressors we experience, the more stressed we feel. It is the experience of something not turning out the way we want it to, largely based on perception and expectations.

Additional Tips

Applying slow deep pressure with a flat palm to large muscles groups can help relieve stress.

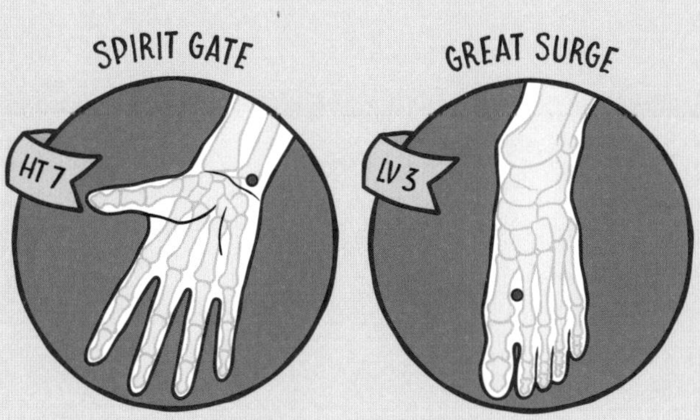

Self-Care

- **Head and Face** routine (see page 118)
- **Neck and Shoulders** routine (see page 119)

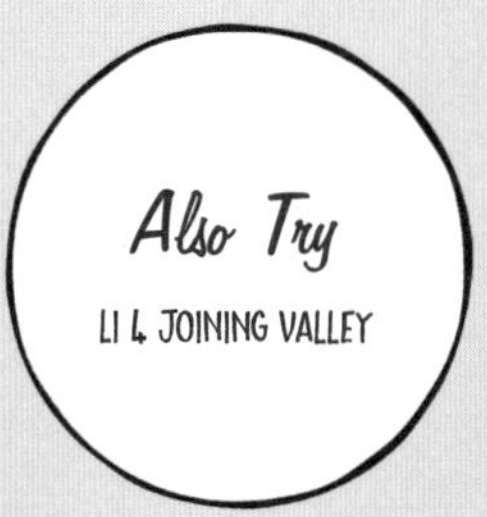

HEAD AND NECK PAIN

Head and neck pain can be due to many factors, including injuries such as whiplash, as well as sleeping with the head in an uncomfortable position, bad posture, headaches, and watching screens for too long.

Additional Tips

Using thumbs or fingers, make small, gentle circles to massage the points shown until the muscle tissue begins to soften and heat is present.

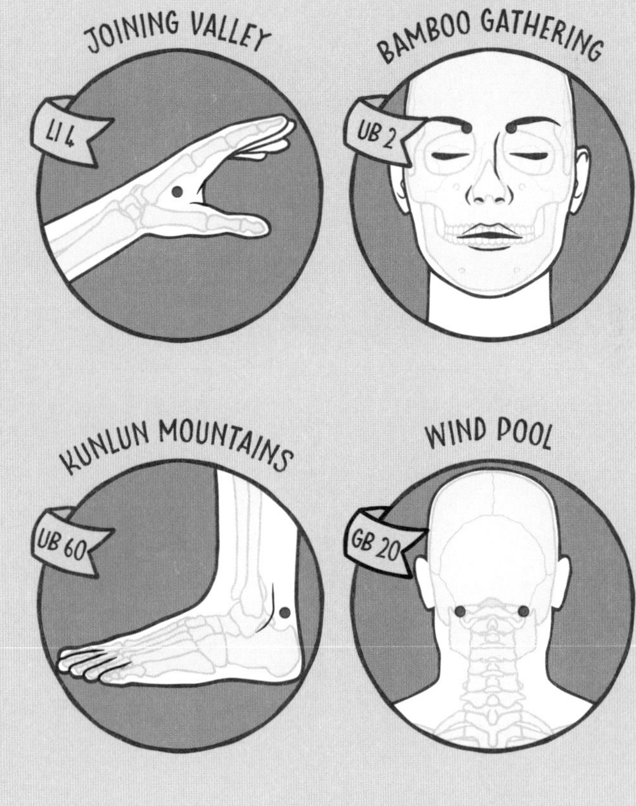

Self-Care

- **Head and Face** routine (see page 118)
- **Neck and Shoulders** routine (see page 119)

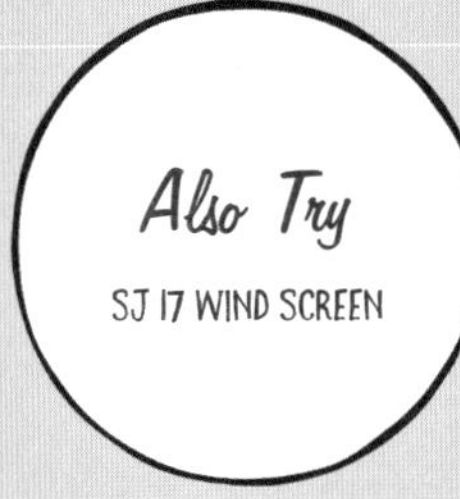

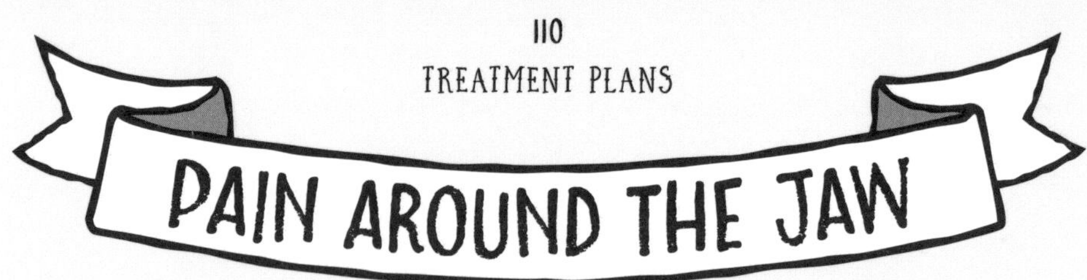

PAIN AROUND THE JAW

There are myriad reasons why a person might experience jaw pain. Some of the most common include TMJD (temporomandibular joint disorder), toothache, and referred pain from either the head/face or neck.

Additional Tips

Using thumbs or fingers, make small, gentle circles to massage the points shown until the muscle tissue begins to soften and heat is present.

Self-Care

- **Head and Face** routine (see page 118)
- **Neck and Shoulders** routine (see page 119)

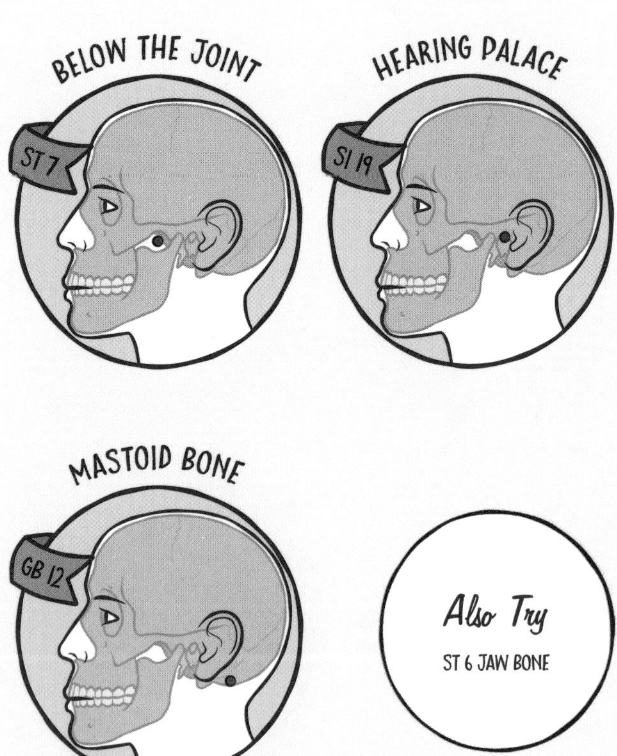

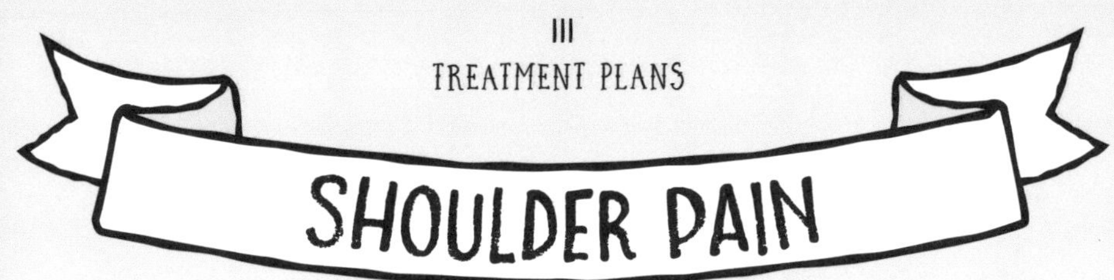

SHOULDER PAIN

Shoulder pain is typically described as any pain or discomfort extending from the base of the head, across the pectoral muscles, around the back over the scapula, to the insertion of the deltoid muscle. Most often this pain is due to improper sleeping positions and repetitive stress from sports activities.

Additional Tips

Using thumbs or fingers, make small, gentle circles to massage the points shown until the muscle tissue begins to soften and heat is present.

Self-Care

- **Neck and Shoulders** routine (see page 119)

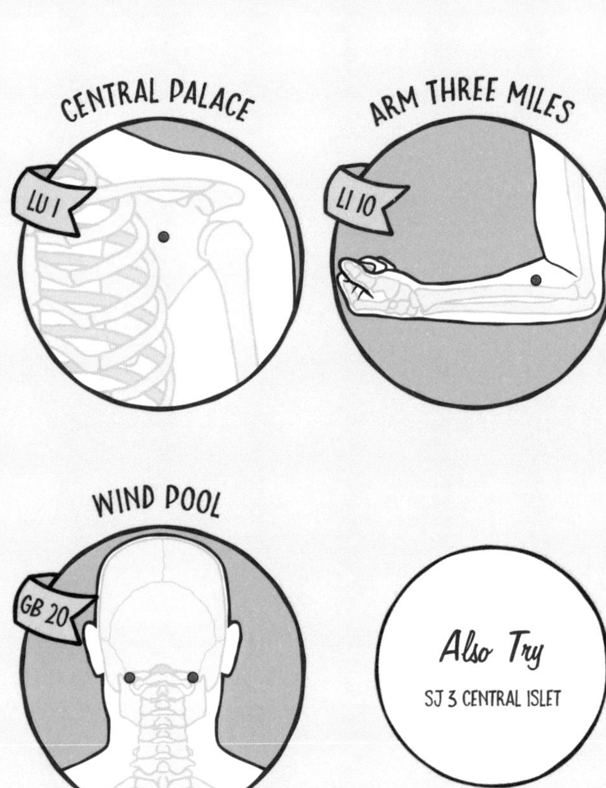

PAIN AROUND THE ELBOW

Elbow pain is considered to be any discomfort around either side of the elbow, including the inside crease. Often, the muscles of the forearm are also indicated as needing massage.

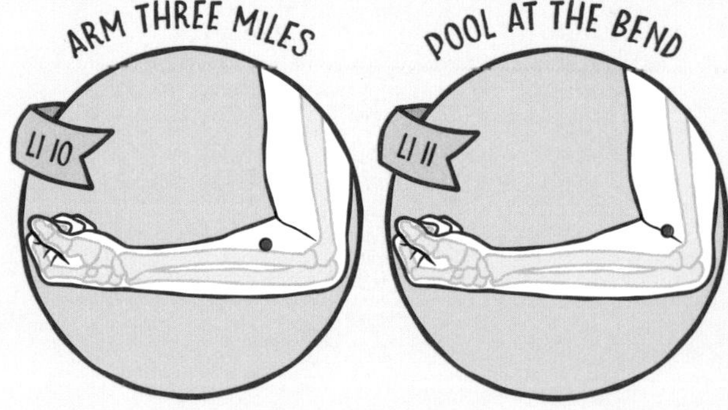

Additional Tips

Using thumbs or fingers, make small, gentle circles to massage the points shown until the muscle tissue begins to soften and heat is present.

Self-Care

- **Neck and Shoulders** routine (see page 119)
- **Arms and Hands** routine (see page 120)

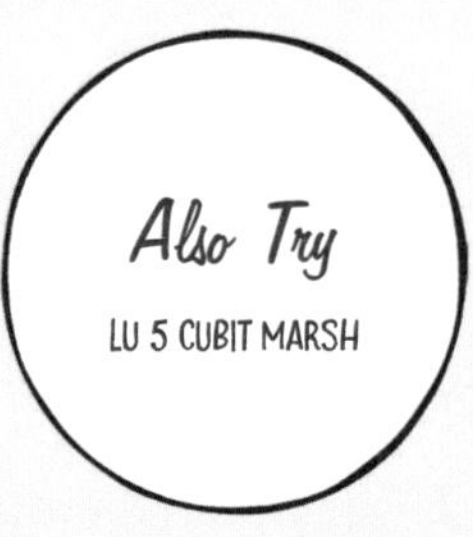

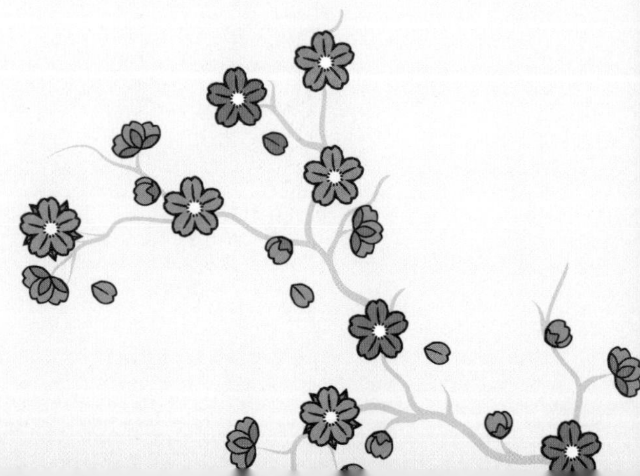

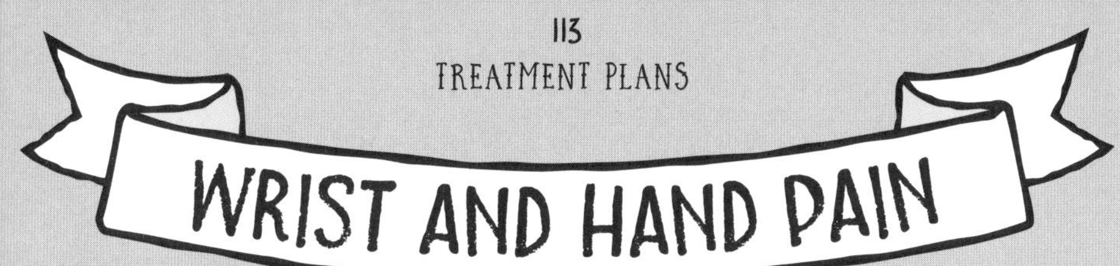

WRIST AND HAND PAIN

Common overuse injuries to the wrist and hand include carpal tunnel syndrome (tingling, numbness, weakness, or pain of the first four fingers and hand), De Quervain's tenosynovitis (inflammation of the tendons and the tendon coverings on the thumb side of the wrist), and general tendinosis (very small micro-tears in the tissue in or around the tendons crossing the wrist and hand).

Additional Tips

Using thumbs or fingers, make small, gentle circles to massage the points shown until the muscle tissue begins to soften and heat is present.

Self-Care

- **Arms and Hands** routine (see page 120)

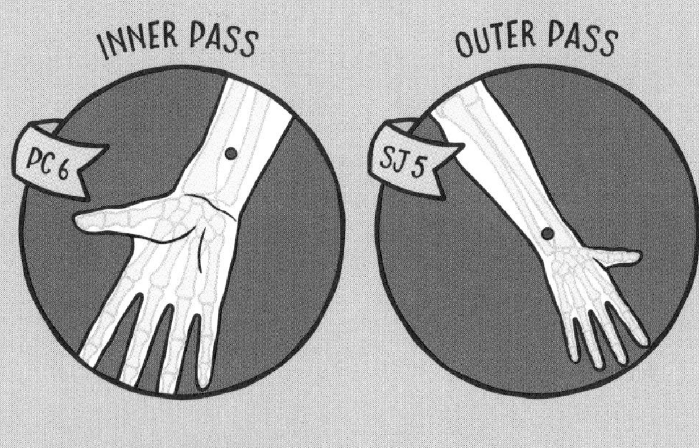

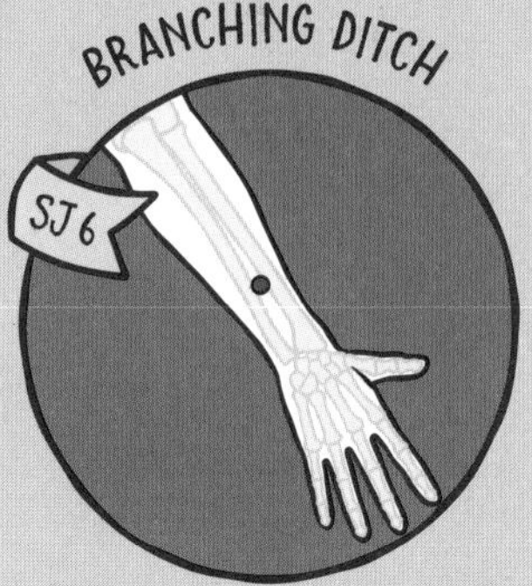

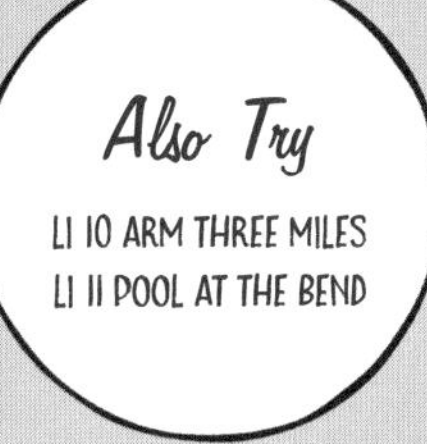
Also Try
LI 10 ARM THREE MILES
LI 11 POOL AT THE BEND

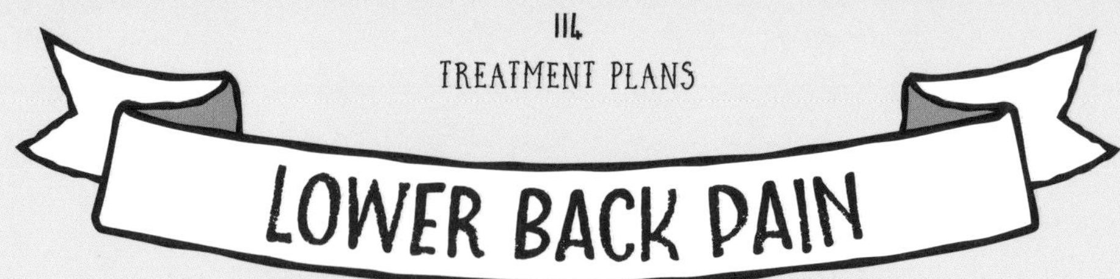

LOWER BACK PAIN

Lower back pain is considered to be any sort of pain or discomfort in the lumbar region, including pain or discomfort when sitting, standing, bending over, stretching, etc. Pain is often described as either a shooting/stabbing pain, or general dull achiness.

Additional Tips

Using thumbs or fingers, make small, gentle circles to massage the points shown until the muscle tissue begins to soften and heat is present.

Self-Care

- **Lower Back** routine (see page 122)
- **Legs and Feet** routine (see page 123)

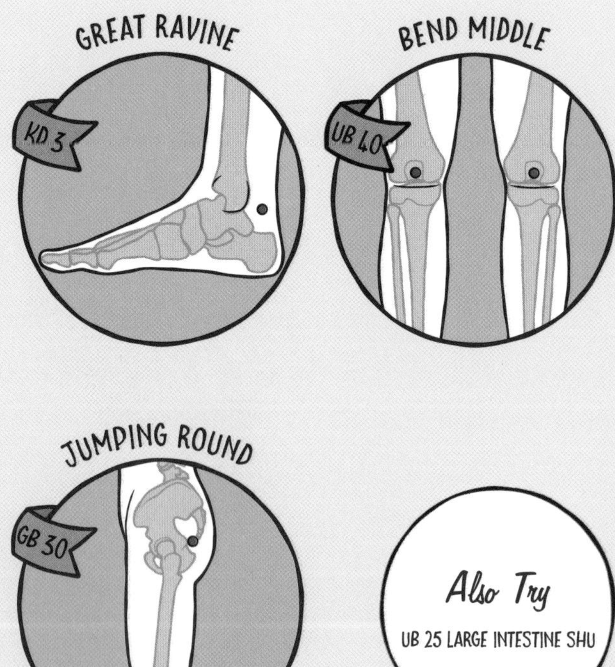

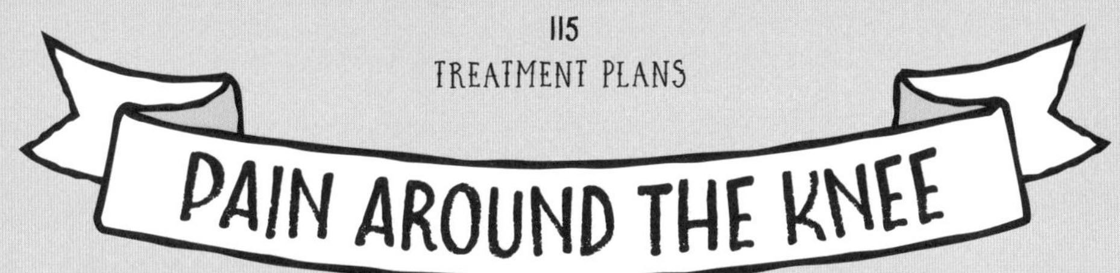

PAIN AROUND THE KNEE

Knee pain may be the result of a number of pathologies, including, but not limited to, meniscus tears, bursitis, patellar tracking syndrome (patella tracking either right or left), chondromalacia patella (breakdown of cartilage under patella), and ACL/MCL (ligament) tears.

Additional Tips

Using thumbs or fingers, make small, gentle circles to massage the points shown until the muscle tissue begins to soften and heat is present.

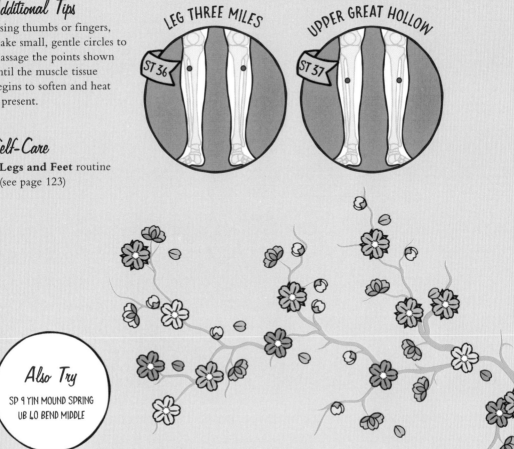

LEG THREE MILES

ST 36

UPPER GREAT HOLLOW

ST 37

Self-Care

- **Legs and Feet** routine (see page 123)

Also Try

SP 9 YIN MOUND SPRING

UB 40 BEND MIDDLE

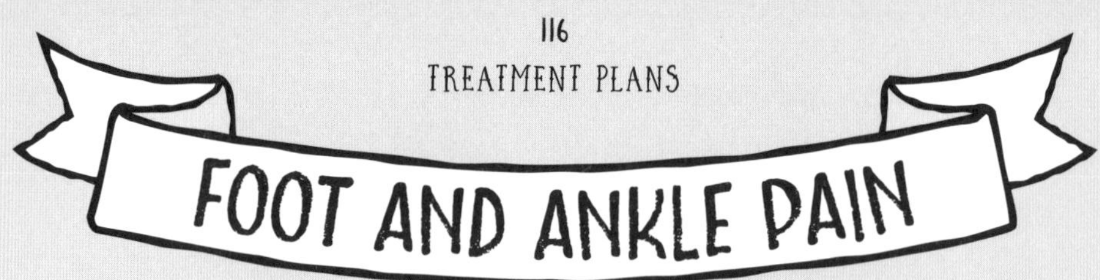

FOOT AND ANKLE PAIN

Common conditions associated with ankle and foot pain may be sprains, strains, injuries, arthritis, and plantar fasciitis.

Additional Tips

Using thumbs or fingers, make small, gentle circles to massage the points shown until the muscle tissue begins to soften and heat is present.

Self-Care

- **Legs and Feet** routine (see page 123)

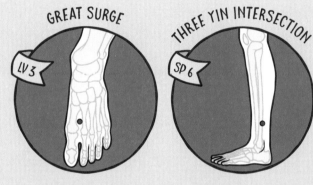

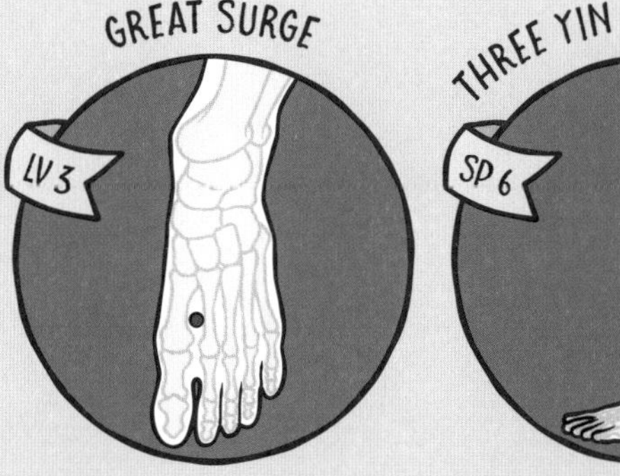

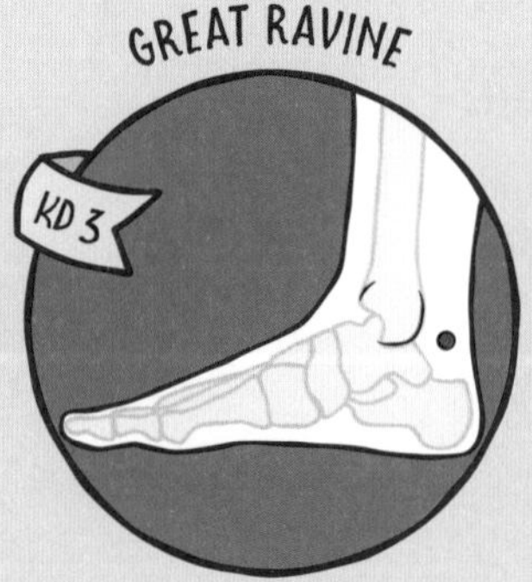

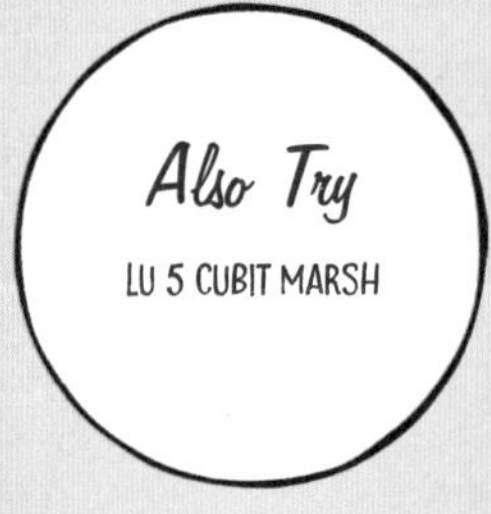

5 THE ROUTINES

He who has health, has hope.
And he who has hope, has everything.

BENJAMIN FRANKLIN

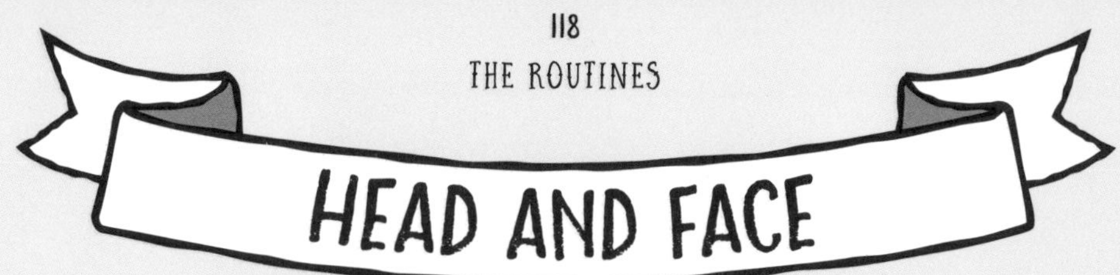

HEAD AND FACE

Working the head and face can seem intimidating at first, especially when treating someone other than yourself. Fear not! Face and head work is considered by the majority of receivers to be the best part of some treatments. Approach with care and confidence, and you will do fine.

HEAD AND SCALP

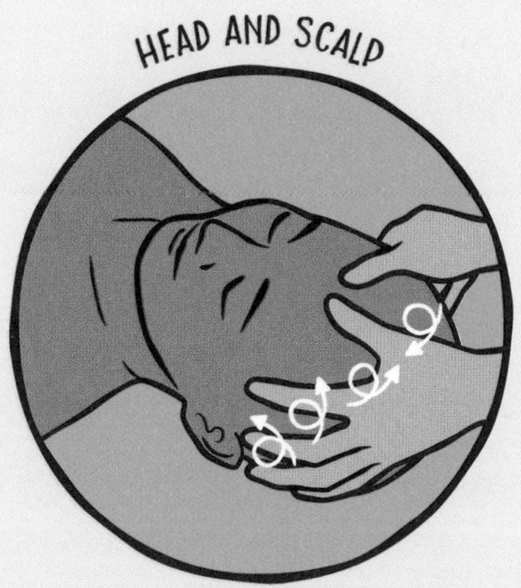

With spread fingers, apply pressure while making circles from the base of the head, above the ears, and toward the crown of the head.

FOREHEAD

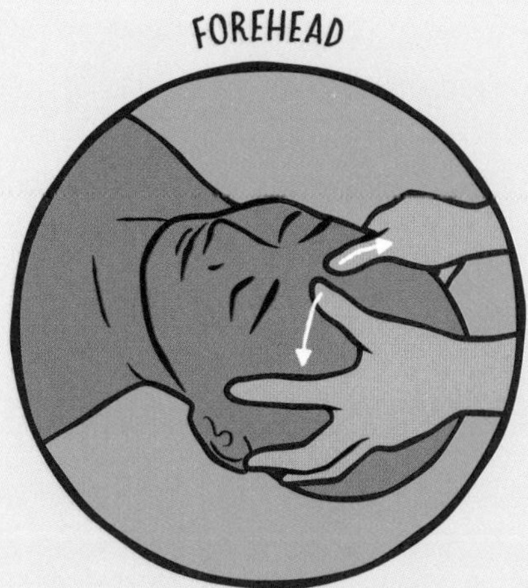

With the pads of the thumbs, make soft, wiping strokes from the center of the forehead outward (above). Finish by placing cupped palms on the head and then over the eyes.

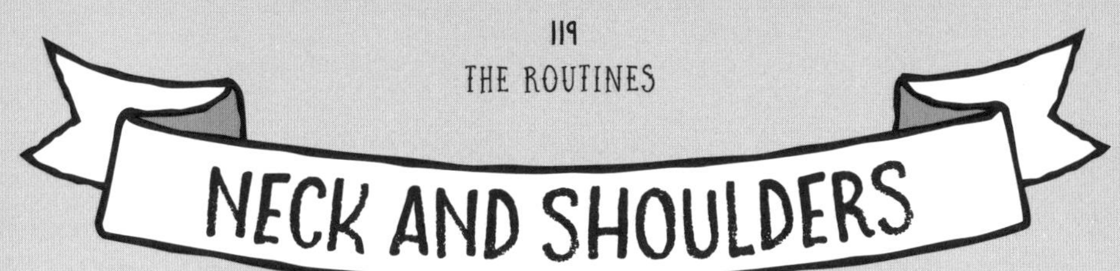

NECK AND SHOULDERS

For many people the neck and shoulders are storage facilities of unrelieved tension. Energetic stasis, as well as muscle tightness, in this area can lead to headaches, along with general feelings of fatigue and irritability.

NECK

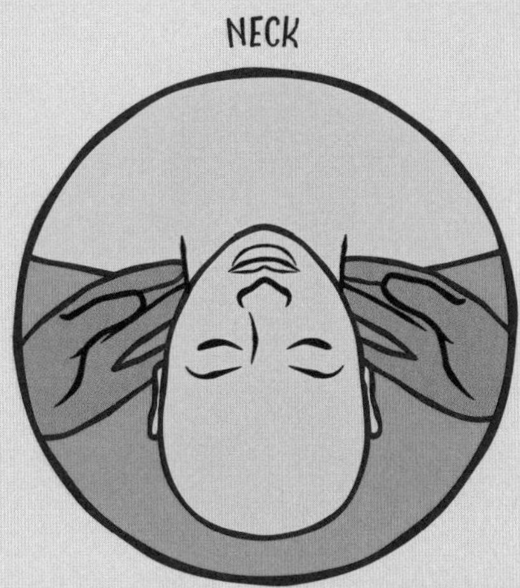

Bring the index, middle, and ring fingers into a point and apply pressure to the upper trapezius muscles. This may also be done with loose fists.

SHOULDERS

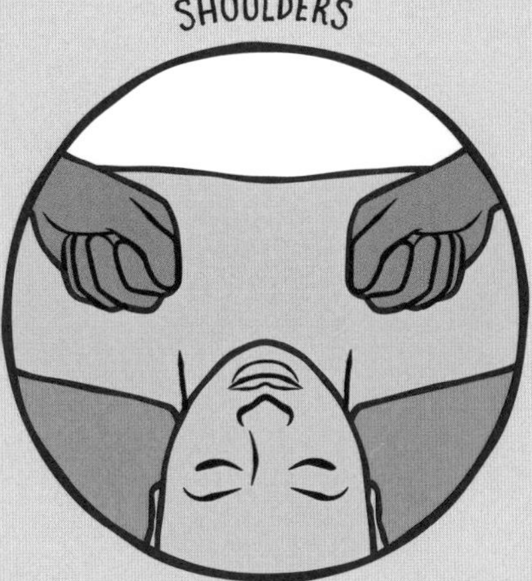

With loose fists, gently press into the cavity near the pectoralis muscles, just below the upper bone of the shoulder.

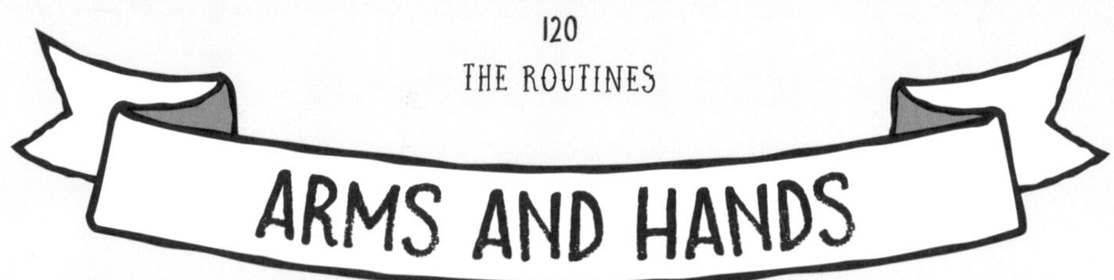

ARMS AND HANDS

Forearms and hands are some of the least worked parts of the body, and yet, especially in our technological age, we use them constantly! Anyone who texts, types, draws, works in manual labor professions, and/or performs acupressure(!) needs this work.

FOREARMS

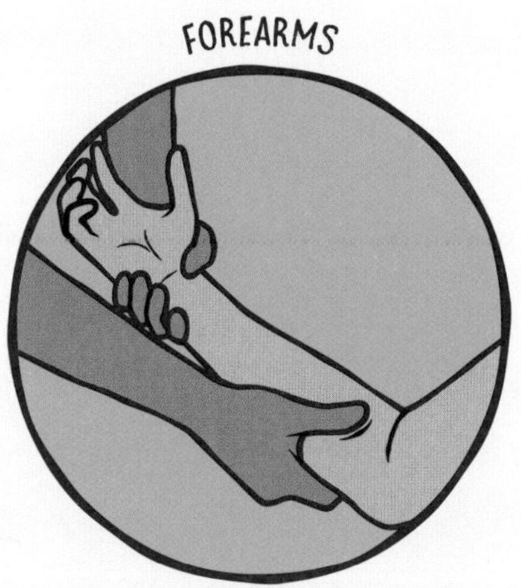

With the arm on its side, thumb facing up, grasp and knead the muscle tissue all along the forearm, paying special attention to the fleshy areas just below the elbow. If there are particularly tender areas in this vicinity (feel around the inner and outer portions of the flesh below the elbow), you may apply gentle, but firm, static pressure to these points.

HANDS

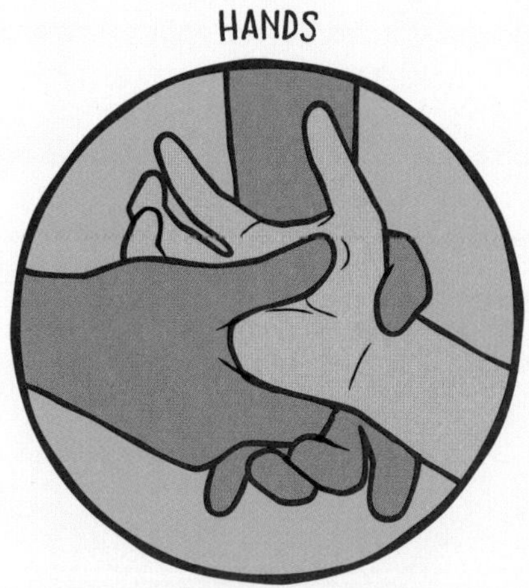

Using your thumbs, press into the fleshy mounds at the root of the hand, making small circles to massage until the muscle tissue begins to soften and heat is present. If there are particularly tender areas (and there usually are!), you may apply gentle, but firm, static pressure to these points.

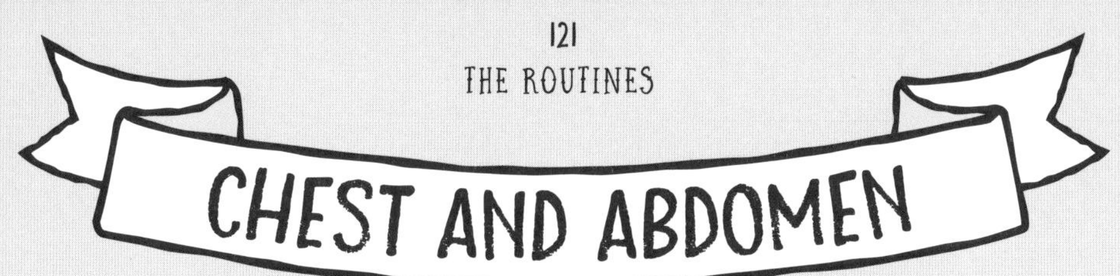

CHEST AND ABDOMEN

So much of what we take in from the world (air, germs, food, liquids) is processed and distributed in the chest and abdomen. A congested chest loves gentle pressure and the wrapping of a loose fist, while a disturbed abdomen benefits from slow, warming strokes.

CHEST

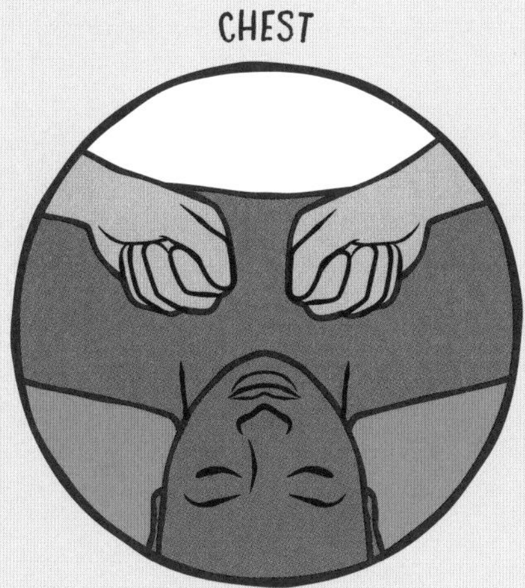

With loose fists, gently press into the cavity near the pectoralis muscles, just below the upper bone of the shoulder. Once the area feels warm, slowly "walk" the fists in place like a cat pawing at the carpet.

ABDOMEN

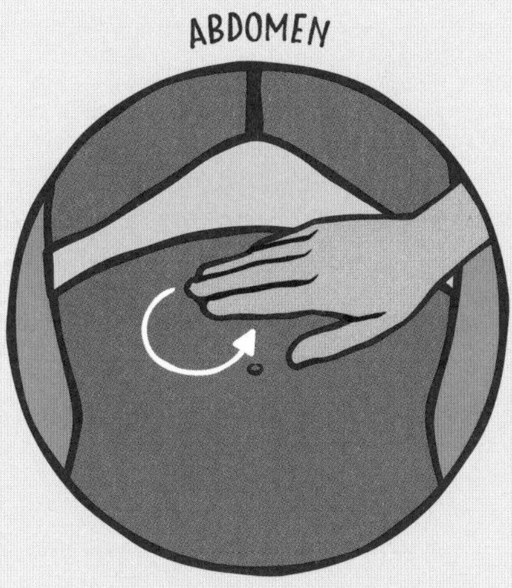

Make slow, warming, circular strokes with a flat palm on the abdomen in a clockwise direction.

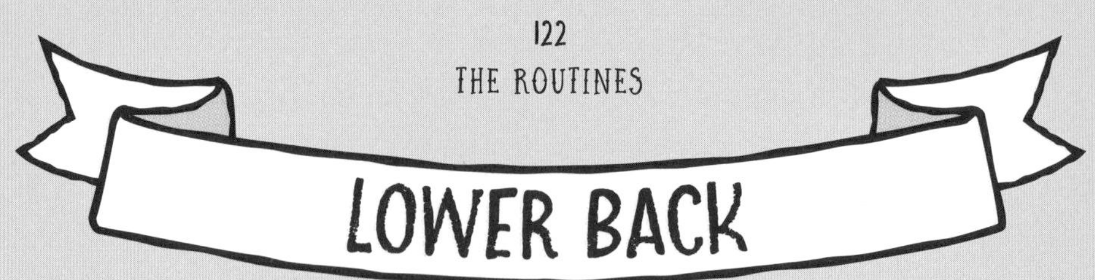

LOWER BACK

Approach this area with care, some warm oil, and long, slow strokes and stretches, and you will have a happy receiver.

LOWER BACK STROKES

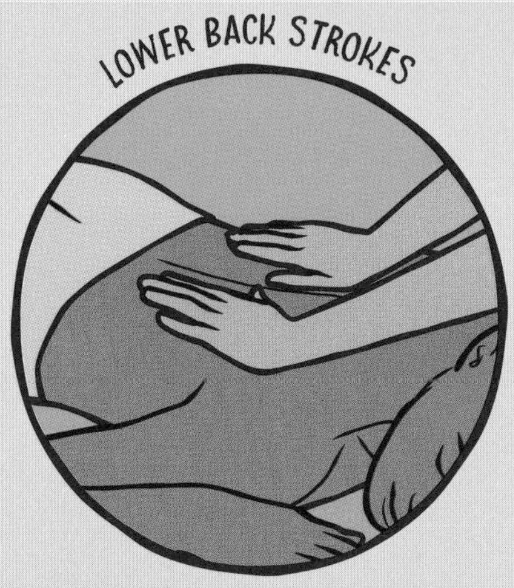

Apply a small amount of lotion to the lower back alongside the spine (not on the spine), and begin long, slow strokes toward the hips.

LOWER BACK STRETCHING

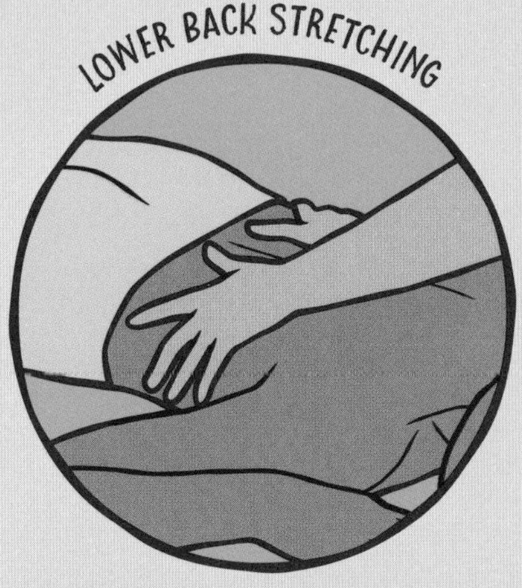

Sitting alongside the receiver, press the heel of the palms on the opposite side of the spine into the muscles of the lower back, pressing the muscles away from the midline. Repeat on the other side.

HIPS

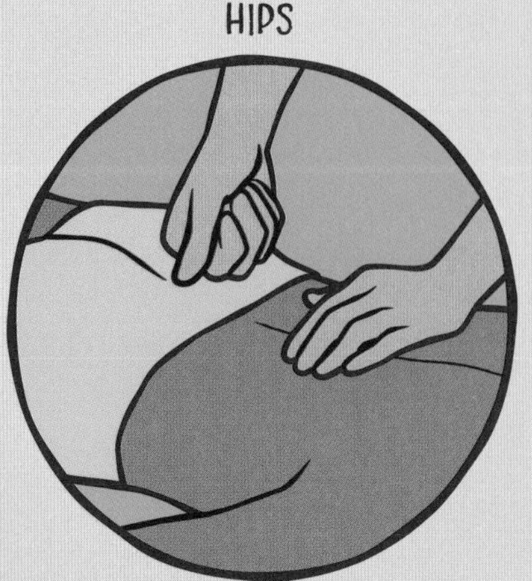

After the lower back becomes warm, press loose fists into the flesh just below the upper bones of the pelvis. Apply direct pressure and hold for one to three breaths. Next, slowly "walk" the loose fists in place to further loosen the tissue.

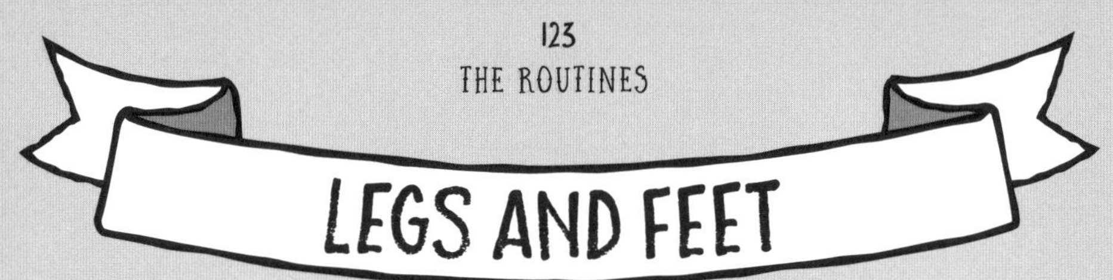

LEGS AND FEET

Sore calves love to be squeezed and massaged, while an angry foot will take all the acute pressure you can give. As always, be mindful of pressure.

CALVES

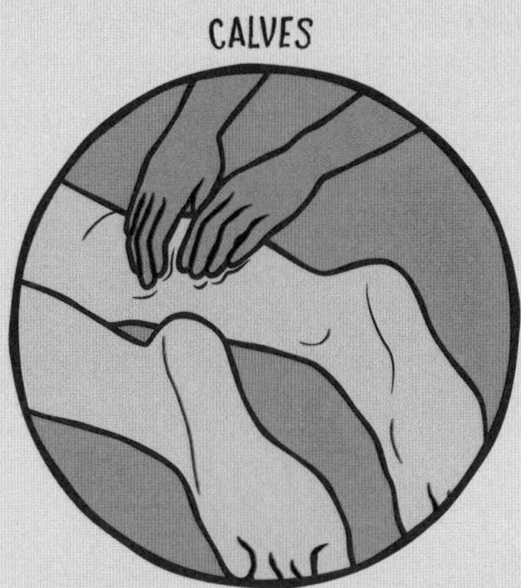

With the receiver face down, fully grasp the flesh of the calves and knead the muscle tissue until it becomes warm. You may also apply static pressure with a flat palm to the calf muscles for one to three breaths.

FEET

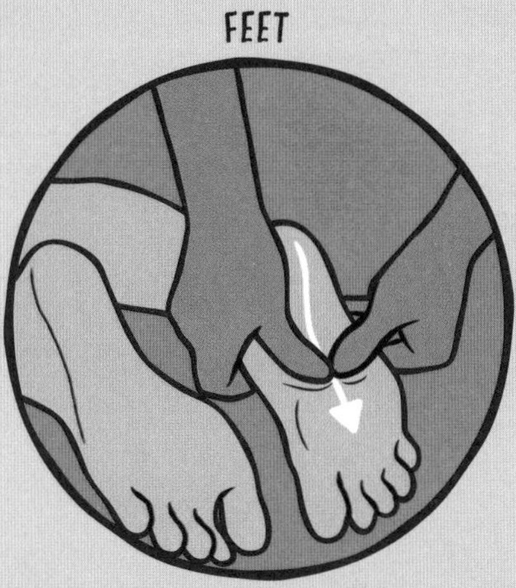

Press thumbs into the sole of the foot and "walk" them from the heel to the ball of the foot.

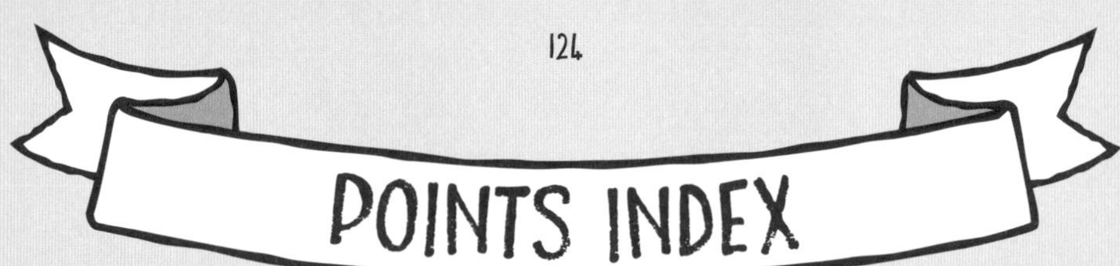

POINTS INDEX

POINTS INDEX

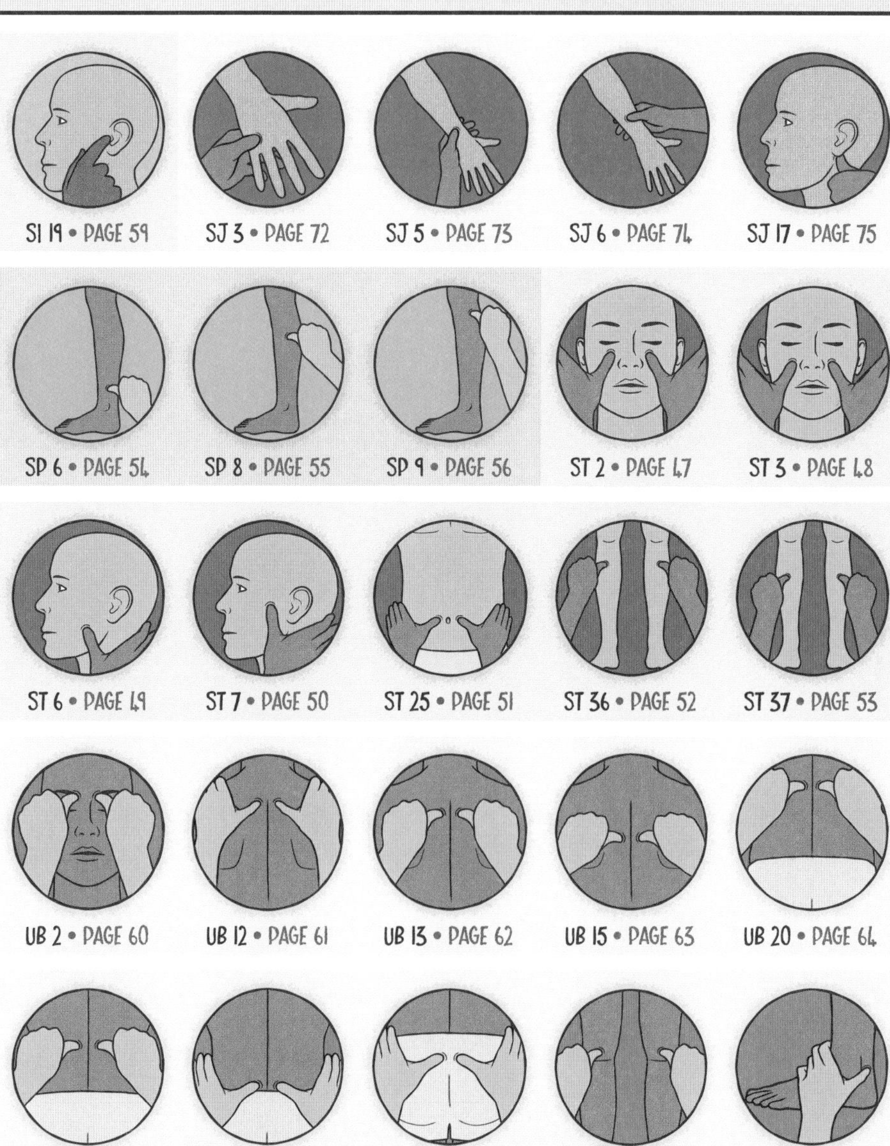

INDEX

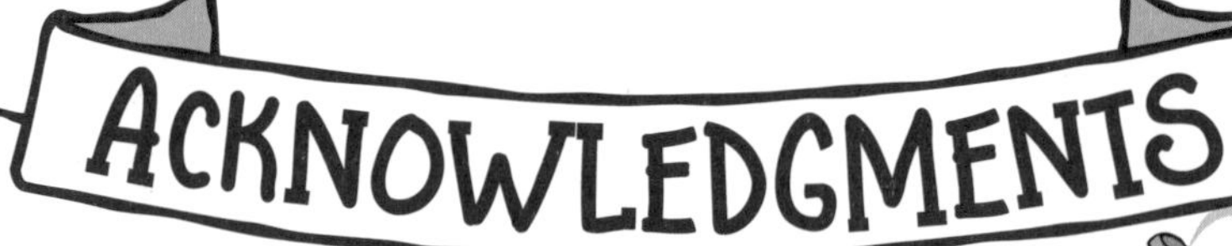

I WOULD LIKE TO FIRST THANK MY TUI NA MENTOR, ERROL LYNCH, HIS TEAM PARTNER, MARIANA ARANDO, AND EVERYONE AT TOUCH TUINA (WHO YOU SHOULD VISIT FOR TREATMENTS IF YOU ARE EVER IN LONDON), FOR THEIR INSPIRATION AND INSTRUCTION. A BIG THANK YOU TO MY FIRST TRUE YOGA INSTRUCTOR, EDDIE STERN, FOR SHOWING ME HOW THE USE OF ACUPRESSURE POINTS CAN BE SO EFFECTIVE IN ALLEVIATING FEAR IN HEADSTANDS, WHICH ULTIMATELY LEAD TO MY BECOMING A MASSAGE THERAPIST. MANY THANKS TO MY INSTRUCTORS AT THE PACIFIC COLLEGE OF ORIENTAL MEDICINE WHO ARE NOT ONLY AMAZING TEACHERS, BUT FANTASTIC PRACTITIONERS. THANK YOU TO MY STUDENTS FOR THEIR HARD WORK AND CHALLENGING QUESTIONS, MY CLIENTS FOR THEIR COMMITMENT TO WELLNESS, MY FRIENDS FOR LETTING ME PRACTICE ON THEM AND NOT SQUIRMING TOO MUCH, AND ESPECIALLY MY FAMILY, WHO SUPPORTED ME, AND HELPED MAKE MY EDUCATION POSSIBLE.

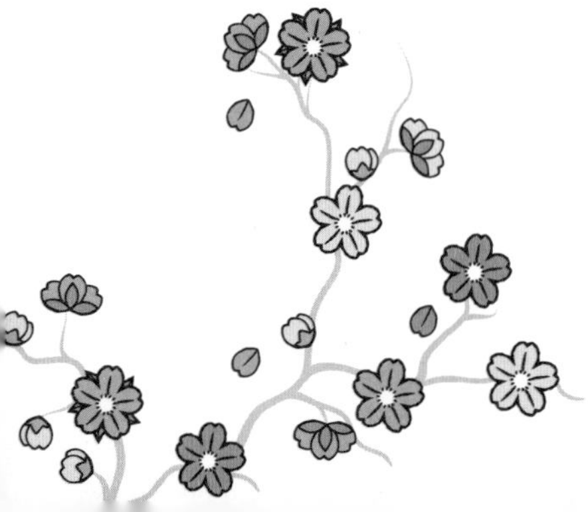